THE NEGOTIATION OF URGENCY

MEDICAL ANTHROPOLOGY: HEALTH, INEQUALITY, AND SOCIAL JUSTICE

Series editor: Lenore Manderson

Books in the Medical Anthropology series are concerned with social patterns of and social responses to ill-health, disease, and suffering and how social exclusion and social justice shape health and healing outcomes. The series is designed to reflect the diversity of contemporary medical anthropological research and writing and will offer scholars a forum to publish work that showcases the theoretical sophistication, methodological soundness, and ethnographic richness of the field.

Books in the series may include studies on the organization and movement of peoples, technologies, and treatments, how inequalities pattern access to these, and how individuals, communities, and states respond to various assaults on well-being, including from illness, disaster, and violence.

For a complete list of titles in the series, please see the last page of this book.

THE NEGOTIATION OF URGENCY

Economies of Attention in an Italian Emergency Room

MIRKO PASQUINI

RUTGERS UNIVERSITY PRESS
New Brunswick, Camden, and Newark, New Jersey
London and Oxford

Rutgers University Press is a department of Rutgers, The State University of New Jersey, one of the leading public research universities in the nation. By publishing worldwide, it furthers the University's mission of dedication to excellence in teaching, scholarship, research, and clinical care.

Library of Congress Cataloging-in-Publication Data

Names: Pasquini, Mirko, 1991– author.
Title: The negotiation of urgency : economies of attention in an Italian emergency room / Mirko Pasquini.
Description: New Brunswick : Rutgers University Press, [2025] | Series: Medical anthropology | Includes bibliographical references and index.
Identifiers: LCCN 2024046858 | ISBN 9781978836266 (paperback) | ISBN 9781978836273 (hardcover) | ISBN 9781978836280 (epub) | ISBN 9781978836297 (pdf)
Subjects: LCSH: Emergency medical services—Italy—Social aspects. | Triage (Medicine)—Italy. | Medical anthropology.
Classification: LCC RA645.7.I8 P37 2025 | DDC 362.180945—dc23/eng/20250312
LC record available at https://lccn.loc.gov/2024046858

A British Cataloging-in-Publication record for this book is available from the British Library.

rutgersuniversitypress.org

To all the patients, caregivers, and health care professionals who still believe in a just, equitable, universal health care system. And among them, especially, to Fre.

CONTENTS

FOREWORD

LENORE MANDERSON

The Medical Anthropology: Health, Inequality, and Social Justice series is concerned with the diversity of contemporary medical anthropological research and writing. The beauty of ethnography is its capacity through storytelling to make sense of suffering as a social experience and to set it in context. Central to our focus in this series, therefore, is how social structures, political and economic systems, and ideologies shape the likelihood and impact of infections, injuries, bodily ruptures and disease, chronic conditions and disability, treatment and care, and social repair and death.

Health and illness are social facts: the circumstances of maintaining and losing health are always and everywhere shaped by structural, local, and global relations. Social formations and relations, cultures, economies, ecologies, and political organizations all shape experiences of illness, disability, and disadvantage. The authors of the monographs in this series are concerned centrally with health and illness, healing practices, and access to care, but in the different volumes, they highlight the importance of such differences in context as expressed and experienced at individual, household, and wider levels. Health risks and the outcomes of social structures and household economies (for example, health systems factors), as well as national and global politics and economics, shape people's lives. In their accounts of health, inequality, and social justice, the authors move across social circumstances, health conditions, geography, and their intersections and interactions to demonstrate how individuals, communities, and states manage assaults on people's health and well-being.

As medical anthropologists have long illustrated, the relationships between social context and health status are complex. In addressing these questions, the authors in this series showcase the theoretical sophistication, methodological rigor, and empirical richness of the field while expanding a map of illness, social interaction, and institutional life to illustrate the effects of material conditions and social meanings in troubling and surprising ways. The books reflect medical anthropology as a constantly changing field of scholarship, drawing on research in such diverse contexts as residential and virtual communities, clinics, laboratories, and emergency care and public health settings; with service providers, individual healers, and households; and with social bodies, human bodies, biologies, and biographies. While medical anthropology once concentrated on systems of healing, particular diseases, and embodied experiences, today the field has expanded to include environmental disasters, war, science, technology, faith, gender-based violence, and forced migration. Curiosity about the body and its vicissitudes remains a pivot of our work, but our concerns are with the location of bodies in social life and with how social structures, temporal imperatives, and shifting exigencies shape life courses. This dynamic field reflects the ethics of the discipline to address these pressing issues of our time.

As the subtitle of the series indicates, the books center on social exclusion and inclusion, social justice, and repair. The volumes in this series illustrate multiple ways that globalization and national and local inequalities shape health experiences and outcomes across space and how economic, political, and social inequalities influence the likelihood of poor health and its outcomes in different settings. At the same time, social and economic relations enable the institutionalization of poverty: they produce the unequal conditions of everyday life and work and hence powerfully influence who gets sick and who is most likely to survive. The books challenge readers to reflect on suffering, deficit, and despair within families and communities while they also encourage readers to remain alert to resistance and restitution—to consider how people respond to injustices and evade the fissures that might seem to predetermine their lives.

A hospital is a beacon, a center of modern technology, expertise, training, and learning; a site of diagnostics, surveillance, and treatment; a place of intervention, repair, respite, and care for people with illness and injuries. It is a point of access to lifesaving measures and emergency interventions. It is also a place of fear—there is always a likelihood that someone presenting for care might die, for why would they present otherwise?—and so it is also a setting to offset serious illness and, often, to save lives.

The most dramatic face of a hospital, in television serials and as witnessed from the street, is the emergency room (ER) or casualty department. Ambulances approach with lights flashing; paramedics urgently brief nursing and other staff; distraught family members hover on the periphery; tangles of leads and tubes for heart monitors and drips camouflage bodies on stretchers; helicopter blades beat out emergency. In such scenarios, some lives are always precarious.

But ERs and casualty departments are also places for reassurance, review, and last resort; as outpatient departments, they meet requests for less urgent attention. Some people present with mundane health problems; some seek diagnostic clarity or want second opinions; others need attention because they lack identity papers, are unemployed, are disturbed, live alone, or lack adequate shelter. For some, the ER is the only place they can afford to seek medical advice and possible treatment.

More than half of the global population lacks access even to basic essential health care, and universal health coverage is elusive. Worldwide, the public hospital system offers people free or low-cost care, including outside the fixed hours of government clinics. People without financial resources, networks, or care systems in place can access family physicians (general practitioners), nurses, midwives, dentists, or others without the extended waiting time necessary at a community health clinic or the cash required to attend a private practice. Open twenty-four hours a day, emergency departments offer care to those not covered for essential health and medical services and those excluded because they lack identity papers, have no money, or have nowhere else to turn. For poor people especially, everywhere, hospital emergency and outpatient departments are the one place where they can receive medical attention. In *The Negotiation of Urgency: Economies of Attention in an Italian Emergency Room* Mirko Pasquini illustrates how this unfolds in urban Italy.

In the face of different demands and requests for care, the triage nurse in an emergency department has a unique task—to categorize need and urgency and so to prioritize the order in which patients may receive attention. In the hospital that Mirko Pasquini describes, the triage nurse evaluates the person who presents in terms of multiple clinical and social signs. Did someone bring them in—a police officer, a family member or a neighbor, a paramedic, or did they present of their own accord? Are they bleeding or struggling to breathe or in acute pain or visibly distressed? Are there other serious clinical signs? Were they brought in following an accident at home? Was there sudden faintness or vomiting? Were they subject to violent attack? And if they regularly visit the department, is this visit any different, or have they presented because—as is the case for some—they have nowhere else to go? How patients are assessed against these questions shapes whether they are ranked as red—a clinical emergency, requiring immediate attention; yellow—urgent, to be seen by a doctor as soon as possible; green—a delayed waiting time; or white—hours spent waiting, with a charge for attention.

Because the triage code shapes how long a person has to wait and the costs of care to them in terms of time, cash, and anxiety, people try to manage how they are perceived by the triage nurse by performing need. Through Pasquini's brilliant and engaging writing, we witness people as they hover by the triage station, as they cry, scream, rage, threaten, and occasionally hit attending staff. They demand stretchers to sleep on and seek examinations (ultrasounds, X-rays, electrocardiograms), specialist consultations, painkillers, and other drugs; crucially—as we read—they demand the attention of health care providers. In interrogating the performance of need and the provision of care, and its scarcity, Mirko Pasquini writes of "economies of attention." These shape how urgency is defined (and refined), how attention is rationed, and how the ER operates through rules, paperwork, structures, and relationships. Urgency, Pasquini writes, is "an unsteady, negotiated, evanescent, and vulnerable accomplishment."

In this compelling account of a seemingly confined space, we learn, too, how the ER reflects the inequalities that shape Italian society beyond its walls. As the Italian welfare state withers and ideas of neoliberalism dominate who might receive attention, why, and when, we see how political economic factors, structural inequalities, austerity measures, and fiscal policies shape the health system and influence the kind of care that might be provided.

Those who present to the ER with vague needs—because they are lonely, cold, poor, or confused, for example, like many of the people of whom we read— sometimes receive little attention, or must wait for it, for their diagnoses do not generate funds to the hospital. As Pasquini explains, because the ER is focused on risk assessment and not on producing diagnoses, it is a "financial sinkhole." Yet the ER's underfinancing is balanced by a greater profit to the hospital as a whole, as many move through the ER to another ward for diagnosis and care. Others are sent away disappointed or frustrated. ER staff, too, are frustrated and bitter, even while struggling to make a difference in the lives and life outcomes of those who seek attention.

The Negotiation of Urgency is a profoundly thoughtful and troubling book. The ER is critical to how a hospital functions, yet it is understaffed and underfunded in this example in Italy, and in general. It is an area of low prestige and high stress, in which patients are often hostile, as much from frustration as pain or fear, and staff are resentful, both from overwork and in reaction to patient hostility. The book tells a deeply familiar story, regardless of the circumstances in which we have presented for care and sat until it is our turn for attention. Mirko Pasquini weaves a powerful story of the people who seek care from the ER, of those who work there, and of the motivations of both. In *The Negotiation of Urgency* he unveils, too, through a lens on the ER, the social, professional, and economic costs of inadequate health systems and the challenges of redressing the neglect that leaves many people with no option but to present and perform their need.

THE NEGOTIATION OF URGENCY

1 · URGENCY AT STAKE

A muscular man in his late thirties, a leather biker's jacket draped over one arm and lavish black tribal tattoos displayed on the other, strides with a swoosh through the sliding glass doors of the emergency room (ER) entrance. It is a crowded, freezing Monday morning in late January. The man plants himself in the middle of the waiting area—a large barren room with eighty plastic seats, garishly lit by neon lights and painted a pale institutional green. He waves a broken glass bottleneck in his right hand, glares in the direction of the nurses' reception area across the room, and shouts, "I want to see a psychiatrist right now, or I'm going to slit my wrists!"

Instead of alarm, this threat is greeted with jaded good humor. The tattooed man, a regular visitor to the ER, is well-known to the staff on duty. "Go on, do it!" Nurse Giovanni—a gruff professional who that morning is seated at the reception desk typing another patient's name and symptoms into his computer—hollers back through the thick glass wall that divides the nurses' reception desk from the external waiting area. "We'll stitch you up. You know we can do it."

The man glares at Nurse Giovanni. "Fine!" he yells. "Then I'll cut my chest open and stab myself in the heart!"

Nurse Giovanni laughs. "Good luck with that! If you can manage to pierce your sternum with a piece of glass, I'll give you a round of applause" (Ti faccio pure l'applauso)!

The tattooed man snorts and looks around, visibly frustrated. Then he turns and strides out through the sliding glass door, as purposefully as he had entered.

During my fieldwork at a large university hospital in northern Italy between 2017 and 2018, I observed signor Valerio,[1] as I later discovered the tattooed man was called, come and go to the ER many times. I became acquainted with his loud shouting and threatening of nurses and doctors. I did not witness the episode with the glass bottle myself; that was recounted to me by Nurse Giovanni with the same vivid, interaction-like storytelling style I report here.[2] I start with this story for the same reason that Nurse Giovanni shared it with me in the first place. This was not solely because it was apparently the only time the man had ever come to the ER armed but because this episode captures what people are capable of doing to gain ER professionals' attention.

Nurse Giovanni knew signor Valerio well enough to conclude that the broken bottle was not intended to hurt anybody. Nurse Giovanni was confident that signor Valerio had caused a scene simply to try to increase the urgency of his demand for help. As I witnessed over and over during my fieldwork, signor Valerio habitually claimed madness in order to skip the long waiting list for primary mental health care. He came to the ER, he once told me himself, because he had an "urgent need to talk to someone" (un bisogno urgente di parlare con qualcuno).

Desperate as his situation was, as he later told me, signor Valerio's was far from an isolated case. Newspapers and television exposés frequently sound the alarm that one-third of the Italian population goes to the ER at least once a year, and 70 percent of those patients are assigned either low-priority or nonurgent care codes (Statistical Portal of the Italian National Agency for Regional Healthcare Services [Portale Statistico AGENAS, n.d.]). In other words, Italian ERs are full of people who the health care staff think do not belong there. Their assumption is backed up by data. From 2012 to 2019, some seven out of ten people examined by nurses and doctors in Italian ERs each year end up being referred to an outpatient facility or are sent home (Portale Statistico AGENAS, n.d.). According to ER professionals, the presentation of people like signor Valerio to the ER, and the demand that this places on services, can be avoided. People like signor Valerio are officially named *utenti impropri*, inappropriate users of the ER.

These people seek different kinds of care in the ER. They include elderly people who suffer from chronic conditions, primarily from noncommunicable diseases. They include undocumented migrants who, only partially covered by national health care insurance, go to the ER for basic health care, such as medication for headaches or colds and routine checkups. Young people who work tight shifts or are struggling to survive the relatively newly restructured Italian neoliberal job market come to the ER to unburden themselves of the mental health problems they face. Some individuals go because they are tired of the lengthy waiting times to get appointments at general health clinics. Others attend because they are lonely and want some kind of social interaction.

The increasing requests for help affect hospital budgets, of which ERs constitute up to 5 percent of total expenditures. In turn, hospitals make up almost half, 44 percent, of Italy's yearly health care budget (Portale Statistico AGENAS, n.d.). The skyrocketing numbers and overcrowding of ERs create a health care crisis of enormous proportion.

Italy is not alone in this situation. ER overcrowding has been an international subject of debate in public health and medical sociology for the last fifty years.[3] In 2011 around 36 percent of patients in ERs in the United States were considered nonurgent (Pines et al. 2011). The numbers are similar in Europe, with rates of between 15 percent in the United Kingdom (O'Keeffe et al. 2018) and 50 percent in Germany (Scherer et al. 2017).

Rather than addressing the so-called inappropriate use of emergency services as a matter of individual responsibility, in this book I address ER overcrowding as a structural phenomenon. I illustrate how ER overcrowding in Italy, as elsewhere, is a direct consequence of policies dictated by the neoliberal principle for which state welfare interventions should be limited, as much as possible, to enhance market competition, considered a primary asset for economic and democratic development. Such rationality of government, a *governmentality* in the words of the French historian Michel Foucault (1991b), places responsibility on individuals rather than on states to take care of people's basic needs, like the one expressed by signor Valerio, who needed a psychiatrist to talk to.

Governmentality, according to Foucault, is a modality of power created by the daily action of key societal institutions redistributing, or denying, care to those in need. Schools, prisons, social services, and, above all, hospitals are institutions where the provision or denial of care can be used as a means of surveillance. This surveillance can either reward or punish individuals and can shape their behavior, effectively turning them into subjects of the state (Foucault 1991b).

For instance, a governmentality that follows the neoliberal principle for which the free market is a primary social good consists of fostering people's subjectivity as health care consumers, rather than as citizens with the universal right to health care. This kind of governance was pursued in Italy by allowing private practices to gain a competitive advantage over public infrastructures by cutting funds for the Servizio Sanitario Nazionale (National Health Service) of about €37 billion (about $45 billion) in the years from the 2008 economic crisis until 2019 (2010–2019, GIMBE Foundation). To guide people's demand for help toward private health care, Italian health care expenditure was reduced by 2019 to 6.2 percent of the gross domestic product, below the average rate in Organization for Economic Co-operation and Development (OECD) countries of 9.5 percent (OECD Health Spending, n.d.).

The cuts were broadly applied, and they hit Italian ERs particularly hard. The national hiring freeze imposed in 2012, and still in force today in 2024, made the historical situation of understaffing in ERs worse than ever. Up to 20 percent of ER shifts, with wide regional differences across the country, are covered by staff hired through private intermediaries (in Italian, *cooperative*, literally "cooperatives") to outsource services and maintain professionals under precarious working contracts, usually lasting only a few months.

Nurses and medical specialists such as psychiatrists were particularly affected by budget cuts and have become increasingly scarce. Short of about 30,000 physicians, 70,000 nurses, and 100,000 hospital beds nationwide, waiting lists for specialist consultations, blood tests or X-rays, or admission to hospital wards by

2010 were so long that people had to wait weeks or even months. Between 2018 and 2019, the average waiting time to see a neurologist or cardiologist was over six months. By 2019 even to see an oncologist and access appropriate oncology tests took more than five months in the public system (Maciocco 2019). While private practices have flourished since 2008, the National Health Service has shrunk in terms of staff, services, and resources (Costa et al. 2016). Underfunded, the national public system is now inadequate to meet the increasingly chronic needs of people in Italy.

The irony—the tragedy—is that as the national health service has shrunk, individuals who cannot afford to turn to private practitioners or private hospitals, and who are dependent on the national health care system for their medical care needs, have increasingly turned to the ER—a service that is always open and accessible to everybody.

The ER thus became the place where urgency is at stake, caught up and contested by competing ways of governing care for those in need. Urgency in the ER is supposed to fit clinical criteria. Triage is designed to ensure timely treatment for heart attacks and stroke, sudden bleeding that might suggest miscarriage or pain indicating acute appendicitis, or broken bones and head traumas due to car accidents or other forms of violence. The ER is not intended to provide routine health care and social support.

During the past fifteen years, however, this definition of urgency has undergone massive renegotiation in Italy. The ER has become the go-to place to try to get painkillers for chronic pain from gallstones or lower back pain; to obtain a routine medical examination because the person has grown weary of waiting for their general practitioner to respond with an appointment time; to check up on stitches, catheters, and bandages after surgical interventions; to get help with consulting specialists such as psychiatrists; or to spend the night when nowhere else is available. The ER has become a venue that people seek out in an attempt to cope with or at least mitigate conditions of bodily, existential, social, and economic precarity. These forms of precarity, for people like signor Valerio with his broken glass bottle, are urgent too.

The profound invisibility felt by the people who crowd the ER in the attempt to be recognized as entitled to medical care and social services by the Italian state contradicts Foucault's influential theorizing of the clinic as a space of governance. Foucault describes the hospital as a setting where people are under constant surveillance, where a sense of penetrating visibility allows the construction of medical knowledge by mapping out bodies with objective examinations or diagnostic tests such as X-rays, magnetic resonance imaging [MRI], or ultrasounds (1994).

In contrast with Foucault's description of the hospital as a space of visibility, in this book I follow the insight of the anthropologist Alice Street. In her work on biomedicine in unstable places, in her case Papua New Guinea, she describes the hospital as a domain where patients and health professionals experience invisibility and subordination to the state (Street 2014). This awareness produces a strong desire to become visible, recognized as entitled to help in a context where without a search for attention a patient may remain invisible, in a state of abandonment.

I take this a step further to analyze how people's search for visibility in the ER has a structural effect within a neoliberal state context like Italy. People's search for visibility and legitimacy for neglected chronic and social conditions forces the Italian state to care for social issues that the neoliberal state actively seeks to disregard. By altering urgency and reappropriating medical language, the people who crowd the ER are able to change the state welfare policy through improvising new spaces of care in the everyday work of the ER. This was what signor Valerio was trying to do with his broken glass bottle.

To document this change in the governance of need created by subaltern actors, in this book I use the analysis of the circulation of attention in the ER as a heuristic to describe the shifting power dynamics in the determination of urgency.

One of the first things one learns inside an ER is that health care providers consider urgency as a developing process, involving the redistribution of concern and material resources over who and what needs to be attended to first to prevent a given situation from worsening. Urgency is a *process* constantly in the making. It is not a self-evident *state* of things. Even within an emergency setting such as the ER, various grades of urgency need to be determined, and those determinations can be altered, contested, or ignored as conditions develop and change. Urgency is fluid and needs constant work to be produced as priority-making. In the ER that work is undertaken through interactions among health care providers, patients, and their friends and relatives within the dynamic environment of the ward.

The making, challenging, and changing of urgency in the ER is called "triage." The vicissitudes of triage are what this book is about.

TRIAGE AND THE VULNERABLE POLITICS OF LIFE

Triage refers to decisions about urgency. From the French verb *trier*, "to sort" or "to choose," the term "triage" originated in eighteenth-century French military medicine. It was used to denote an assessment technique to classify injured soldiers on the battlefield according to the urgency of their needs in relation to the availability of treatment by emergency services (Iserson and Moskop 2007, 276–277). Who to help live and who to let die, what to attend to first, and how to set priorities—triage is the decision-making process to determine urgency.

Since the World War II, clinical triage has developed in different ways: in humanitarian aid settings (Pandolfi 2003; Fassin and Pandolfi 2010; Redfield 2013);

in prehospital emergency medical services (Seim 2020; Stonington 2020); in intensive care units (Kaufman 2006, 2015); in determining priority for organ transplant (Lock 2002; Sharp 2013); in priority-making in relation to medical preparedness and pandemics (Caduff 2015); and in ERs (Lachenal, Lefève, and Nguyen 2014; Solomon 2022). All these kinds of triage are based on an imbalance between resources to be allocated and demands for help to be addressed. In disaster triage, as occurred during the COVID-19 pandemic, such imbalance is so dire that urgency of treatment is determined according to chances of survival. Individuals judged to have better chances of survival and less risk of dying get treated first.

This logic is generally reversed in an ER, where the imbalance between resources and requests for help is less stark. There, those who are most at risk of rapidly becoming worse and dying, and who have less chance of survival if left untreated, are treated first.

Clinical triage is the first moment in the negotiation of urgency in the ER.[4] Patients first undergo a clinical triage process, and then they see a doctor. Clinical triage is carried out by nurses and is composed of four phases of evaluation that end up assigning each patient with a color code: red (clinical emergency, immediate attendance), yellow (urgent need, brief waiting time to be seen by a doctor), green (low urgency, long waiting time for doctor's examination), and white (nonurgent, longest waiting time to be seen by a doctor).

For patients, these codes—the details of which will become apparent in chapter 3—have consequences in terms of both waiting time and contact fees. For the health care providers who work in the ER, the codes are a practical way to organize workflow and distribute available resources according to people's assessed needs. But even though the criteria for assessment are clearly set out on paper, clinical triage, as part of the larger process of accomplishing urgency in the ER, is a vulnerable project. It requires work to be determined and maintained, and it is subject to changes due to newly emerging conditions, such as a widespread lack of access to care and the existential precarity experienced by an increasingly large proportion of the Italian population.

As presented to the nurses in training and within the medical literature that explains triage, clinical triage is treated largely as a neutral adjudication of fixed categories applied in order to sort people's conditions into different groups (i.e., into who is to receive care first and who needs to wait). Medical anthropologists, on the other hand, have questioned the neutrality of such medical categories. Rather than being regarded as a kind of impartial sorting procedure, in medical anthropology triage is seen as a set of practices that actively create difference by performing "medical ethics and reason" influenced by historically, politically, and socially determined ideologies (Lachenal, Lefève, and Nguyen 2014, 10).[5] Medical anthropologists use "triage" to denote how governmentality is carried out by state institutions, bureaucracy apparatuses, families, and humanitarian interventions (Biehl and Eskerod 2005; Nguyen 2010; Redfield 2013; Solomon 2017, 356).

An example is the anthropologist Vinh Kim Nguyen's research on the HIV epidemic in West Africa. Working with programs of humanitarian aid and examining state and international political responses to the epidemic, Nguyen describes how, during the HIV outbreak in Côte d'Ivoire, triage as a practice of "selecting those who would receive the treatments and those who would not" (in this case antiretroviral drugs) became more than a medical system of sorting (2010, 109). Triage became an instrument of governmentality, a way by which HIV humanitarian aid programs encouraged people to behave like subjects worthy of receiving lifesaving medical treatment (Nguyen 2010).

Triage governs not only life and care but also death and disease. The decision to deny help and create death—the dark side of triage named "necropolitics" by Achille Mbembe (2019)—is increasingly deployed to produce social worth. For instance, the anthropologist João Biehl, in writing of Vita, an asylum for people disregarded by both state and family support in Porto Alegre, Brazil, shows how triage can be used to govern how outcasts, like the people with drug addictions he describes, are allowed to die (Biehl and Eskerod 2005). The story of Biehl's key informant, Catarina, reveals triage as a way of governing people's death by systematically denying them care through the different medical, psychiatric, and family worlds from which they are excluded (Biehl and Eskerod 2005).

Scholars such as Nguyen and Biehl highlight how triage, as a system of adjudication that is historically, politically, and socially determined, reproduces social arrangements by making decisions about who is worthy of attention and care. Those decisions are embedded in, and indicative of, particular understandings of deservedness and moral worth (Fassin 2005, 2015). Triage discloses people's value, revealing who would be publicly grieved when passing away and who would depart silently, without even being mourned (Butler 2006).

Triage, for medical anthropologists, is therefore a tool to govern people's life by distributing or denying them care. By relying on categories portrayed as scientific and neutral, triage is the pinnacle of medical and state authority; it makes politically and morally charged decisions about things like who gets to survive or who first receives care. Such decisions are described as a biopolitics, a politics of life, by Michel Foucault (1998), and they leave deep marks in a context like Italy, characterized by a profound inequality. They shape the way the state, medical services, and people negotiate social worth and value.

But, as I will show, what happens when the governing of care, as a way to create state subjects, does not go as planned? What happens when people in subaltern power positions are capable of creating spaces of exception in which urgency can be dealt with in new terms? Triage itself is subject to changes as a material, and thus vulnerable, care governance project.

The material vulnerability of triage is illustrated by the work of the anthropologist Harris Solomon (2017, 2022) in a casualty ward in Mumbai. Focusing on urban traffic injuries, Solomon details how triage decisions have changed due to the sluggish pace of bureaucratic work in the ward and how road regulations influence clinical decisions about how to deal with car crashes, police questioning, or ensuring transit between hospitals and the impossibility of doing so in rush-hour traffic (2017, 355–358; 2022, 54–78).

Solomon's description of a triage that must be "adjusted" to different settings constitutes an important step toward perceiving triage as a nonfixed, iterative process of making urgency. First, it highlights the possibility for triage and the governing of care to be changed within the context of its application. Second, it frames triage as a process in which multiple parties are simultaneously involved in decision-making. These insights suggest that we might expand the reach of such an analytical frame even further, nuancing "adjustment" by attending to the constant negotiation by which triage is crafted in context, amid diverse actors who stand in asymmetric power relations and who at times hold competing or even openly clashing understandings of what constitutes urgency.

Medical expertise and patients' views clash, sometimes destructively. Mistrust coming from patients and mistrust directed at patients by health care professionals occur in a context of potential violence—both immediate physical violence and verbal violence such as threats of lawsuits. How is medical authority asserted amid relations of suspicion, mistrust, and potential violence? How do different understandings of urgency undergird a potential for violence in the ER? While crucial health care interventions do occur in the ER, what actually happens is subordinated to uncertain or fragmentary information, shifting resources, and unpredictable interactional dynamics. Throughout this book, I show how multiple uncertainties are a structuring feature of urgency in the ER.

By analyzing how urgency is made in the ER, in this book I seek to contribute to the anthropological literature on triage by analyzing it not as an *adjudication*, as the medical literature asserts, or an *adjustment* to movements in space, as Solomon suggests, but rather as a *negotiation* of priorities in practice. This move is significant because it acknowledges the major role that recurring disputes between diverse actors have in determining urgency while also restructuring health care governance within and outside the ER premises.

In addition to sorting people's needs according to clinical assessment and immediate signs of distress or crises, triage in the ER develops practically as a series of ongoing negotiations around limited resources, in situations in which there is a constant tension between, on the one hand, health care providers' efforts to maintain control of their medical authority and decision-making and, on the other, patients' demands for care, which, as I have already suggested, are increasingly linked to societal conditions of precarity.

Among the limited resources under negotiation are stretchers to sleep on, medical staff and technologies for examinations (including ultrasounds, X-rays, electrocardiograms [ECGs]), specialist consultations, painkillers and drugs, and, crucially, the attention of health care providers. In focusing on covert tensions and open conflicts in the ER, I reveal urgency as an unsteady, negotiated, evanescent, and vulnerable accomplishment.

The perspective I develop is that triage is urgency in practice. Urgency is not a fixed category assigned by a single decision-maker. It is the fluid result of interactions between multiple actors within a context of care governance in the ER. It is also constantly vulnerable in the sense that it can be changed, and so it is never fully settled.

To illustrate this, in this book I examine how the attention of health care providers is shaped and reshaped both by situational developments such as, for instance, a patient's changing medical condition or the presence of multiple emergencies and by the desires and demands of individual patients, their family members, and the colleagues of health care professionals.

What I call "economies of attention" is a kind of limbic system that runs through the ER and allows urgency to gel. An economy of attention is a modality of power through which focus is directed and relations are prioritized, in terms of what needs to be attended immediately and what can wait, what is important in a given situation, and what can be left unattended. Such a focus on triage as a constant negotiation of attention contributes, more generally, to the scholarly literature about how life and death in hospitals reflect their resources and constraints.[6]

The changing conditions in which triage in hospitals occurs today are underreported in scholarly work. Those changing conditions became of vital importance as the COVID-19 pandemic unfolded. My fieldwork in the ER was conducted in 2017–2018 and had already concluded by the time the pandemic hit Italy in February 2020. However, the kinds of economies of attention that I explore in the chapters that follow can helpfully address some of the changes triggered by the pandemic. I address them explicitly in the conclusions by drawing from phone interviews, media coverage, and the follow-up fieldwork I conducted among general practitioners between 2021 and 2022.

ECONOMIES OF ATTENTION IN THE ER

In the ER, urgency can be understood as a negotiation around that which requires the most attention. But what is attention?

Attention is here understood as the basic unit of medical care, which well represents its being at once a creative, generative form of power and a surveilling, punishing one. Attention can be understood as, first, a basic relational act of empathy and recognition, a form of openness, of "caring about" others (Petrement 1977; Klaver and Baart 2011). At once, attention is also a selective mechanism, a "spotlight" that may be used as a form of surveillance (James 1950). To "watch over" somebody is to assert control, to determine the boundaries of what is legitimate, what is normal, and what is pathological (Canguilhem 1988).

By the same token, through medical care, state institutions both support citizens' lives by healing and relieving them from suffering while they also watch over their ability to flourish, reproduce, work, and be active members of society. The apex of such a relationship of governance is the decision-making implied in urgency, as the decision over who will access care immediately and who will have to wait.

Attention as shaping, creating, or withdrawing care priorities allows me to analyze how the limited resource of health care providers' attention circulates in the ER and how it is influenced by many things, both small (a patient's demands for opioid drugs to relieve pain) and large (wide-scale conditions of socioeconomic precarity, in the context of health care neoliberalization).

In the ER, the attention of health care professionals determines who will be attended to and who must wait. Attention determines urgency. It is readapted in context and is subject to sudden changes in tasks, resources, and demands from incoming patients, ambulance staff, nurses, and doctors. Attention determines the pace of interactional dynamics, creating temporalities centered around a moving hierarchy of tasks to be foregrounded or backgrounded. But attention is not random or unstructured; it circulates, and its circulation enables the practical work of the ER as a "microphysics" of power (Foucault 1991a, 26). In this book I highlight attention as the basic unit of care, as a spotlight that implies a constant trade-off between what is made visible and what is left out of sight.

Attention constitutes an active counterpart of "visibility," a concept that, beginning with Michel Foucault's "birth of the clinic" argument, has had an impressive uptake in medical anthropology scholarship (1994). Both visibility and attention illustrate two alternative ways to articulate the relationship between power and knowledge in medical encounters. According to Foucault, power expresses its field of exercise in the way knowledge is distributed (1998). Knowledge therefore determines what is at stake and what can be acted upon in intersubjective relationships (Foucault 1998). Foucault's concept of visibility articulates this relation as a passive one.

For instance, the objectification of bodies by the medical gaze draws boundaries and cartographies that reveal ways to act over death and disease. But there is no interaction, nor the possibility for such a relationship between the observer and the observed to be changed. In contrast, attention represents an alternative way to understand the nexus of power and knowledge in dynamic terms. Whereas visibility implies passivity—of a body objectified by the medical gaze—attention is an active resource that can be both bound to medical exigencies and also bent to contextual happenings and people's emerging needs.

As an active resource, attention makes visibility emerge only as a contextual achievement, through the redistribution of concern within interactions between diverse actors. It is never a passive relation that establishes vision once and for all, like the biomedical scrutiny over the body described by Foucault. Attention is thus better able to represent dynamism and change within the node of power and knowledge.

Attention as an analytical and theoretical key offers an additional advantage, that of representing the influence that people in an asymmetrical relationship can wield on structural power change. As I will show, the pressure exerted by overcrowding on the ER, and more generally on the health care and the welfare system, is a clear example of such a dynamic. Revisiting the nexus of power and knowledge described by Foucault, I use attention as a heuristic to describe the redistribution and improvisation of urgent care as a basic resource of state governance toward its citizens.

Using the ER as a window to the outside world, I illustrate what daily life in the ER reveals about the growing inequity in Italy and other countries experiencing an important privatization of their national public health care systems. Italy in particular represents an extreme case in Europe. At the time of my fieldwork, the country was rapidly shifting from a universalistic health care service to a system increasingly based on American-inspired private insurance, which considered the state only as a guarantor for the least profitable essential services, first and foremost the emergency care departments. Italy found itself at the center of a perfect storm in which aging demographics, privatization of the universalistic health care system, and increasingly right-wing-leaning policies met the daily vicissitudes of what is for many the last available public place to receive care and help—the ER. There the effects of state withdrawal from welfare are daily revealed by the conflicts that give rise to the negotiation of urgent care needs within the public emergency service.

In the ER, not only is the urgency granted to people's needs redefined but also people's role as citizens can be redefined. Following Foucault's analysis of governmentality, state power is not mainly exemplified by the making of laws (1991b). Rather, state governance is revealed in the administration of goods, needs, and desires of the population. The governance of care is thus a key context of state formation, one in which the creation of citizens as state subjects is at play (Seim and DiMario 2023). The ER in particular provides a setting to consider the state's capability, or not, to care for situations of often profound desperation. Signor Valerio's efforts for attention in the ER are just one example. The analysis of the different, shifting ways in which attention circulates in the ER can help us explore the practical effects of the changing nature of the welfare state in Italy, as elsewhere.

METHODOLOGICAL CONSIDERATIONS

In my fieldwork, I aimed to immerse myself completely in the rhythm and work of the ER. I was able to do so due to the exceptional freedom that the hospital facility granted me as an ethnographer looking at overcrowding: a longtime problem on which the hospital management was eager to gain a new perspective. My research in the ER was also part of my PhD education in cultural anthropology at Uppsala University. This allowed me to be a full-time "research visitor" (*visitatore ai fini di ricerca*) for a year in the ER.

My fieldwork was thus different from the more traditional "on-call" shadowing or "waiting for a good case" often used to observe interactions within clinical settings.[7] I worked the same entire shifts as the triage nurses I was following, each one from eight to twelve hours.[8] For twelve months, between November 2017 and November 2018, I spent five to six days per week working morning, afternoon, and night shifts. The intensity of this fieldwork allowed me to engage with the vicissitudes of the ER, with its ups and downs, with its alternate waves carrying peaks of quick, contemporaneous events, and with people who were anxiously waiting to be noted and attended to.

My work in the ER altered my way of seeing the world. My notion of risk changed profoundly, as occurrences that many of us are unlikely to ever contemplate become brutal realities in the ER—the tragic explosion of gas ovens or of toilets due to a sudden heightened water pressure, for example, or the incredible danger of simple acts like crossing the road, walking down a flight of stairs, cooking, boiling oil and water, or using sharp cutlery. Witnessing the dire consequences of some of those banal actions made me feel uneasy about everyday life. As the anthropologist Sharon Kaufman (2015) discussed in her work on lifesaving treatments in the United States, in the ER the ordinary meshes garishly with the exceptional. One consequence of this unsettling juxtaposition, for me anyway, was that the ordinary world turned into a much more frightening place.

My presence in the ER generated an interesting tension. I have noted how in the ER there existed a specific economy of attention to set urgency, which was vulnerable to change and needed constant work to be maintained. As someone present in the ER, I was unavoidably part of such an economy of attention. But I was also a persistent glitch in its flow. Particularly at the beginning of my fieldwork, more than once I was gently chastised for ignorantly being in the way of nurses and doctors trying to do their work. It took time for me to learn when and where I could engage professionals with questions about what they were doing and when they needed space to concentrate, when I could follow them closely, and when I should just let nurses and doctors alone with, for instance, a patient whose demands for aid turned suspiciously silent when they saw me and wondered who I might be.

During fieldwork, I participated in creating the economy of attention that constitutes the work of making urgency. I transported stretchers; reassured patients; translated conversations from and into English (for migrants who spoke no Italian); brought blankets, pillows, dry ice, and bandages; acted as a secretary and wrote reports of staff meetings; organized focus groups to rediscuss procedures; fetched medication ordered by the staff; and collected and helped to edit documents, all while running around the ward with health care providers. I was the only person who, wearing a lab coat (which I was obliged to wear in the inner part of the ER for hygiene purposes), shifted between the internal triage area and sitting outside in the external waiting room. Multiple times every day, I crossed the triage "barricade"—that is, the wall of glass that separated the examination rooms from the waiting room.

My position in the ER was divided into two basic methodological moments. First, I shadowed triage nurses and their inpatient procedures, following them around with a notebook and digital recorder. I observed, discussed, and asked for explanations, which most nurses and doctors gladly gave me, treating me like a young nurse or medical student in training. I helped the staff with material assistance such as escorting patients to examination locations, and I assisted with the heavy lifting of patients during medical procedures, as a spare pair of hands. Both nurses and doctors tried to teach me about their clinical work. I learned how to read and do medical examinations of different sorts (e.g., take vital measurements, conduct electrocardiograms, and make clinical evaluations), to memorize guidelines, and to look for diverse practical applications. These were to me the most unfamiliar of things since I was not a trained health care professional—a different native language that took on a life of its own in the ER, both matching and differing from manuals of medical knowledge.

Second, I sat in the external waiting room with patients and caregivers. I provided them with answers to questions like "Where am I on the patients' list?," "Who should I ask about X?," and "What's happening now?" An important part of my work in the ER was to pay attention to the suffering and frustration of both patients and health professionals. Of course, listening and attending to what goes on in people's lives is part of every ethnographer's job. But in the ER, because attention is a scarce resource, it is one of the most important bestowals one may obtain. The time I took to talk to people was generally appreciated and only rarely rebuffed or refused. Semistructured and informal interviews also became a way to listen to people's troubles and offer them a sympathetic ear. I conducted eighty-six interviews inside and outside the ER venues.

I was allowed by many of the patients and triage nurses to audio record their interactions during the triage assessment (ninety-four recordings overall). When I quote speech in the text, it is either because I recorded the interaction/interview or because I noted it down right after. The only case in which I used an approximation is the case of the opening vignette with the tattooed man, which was recounted to me by Nurse Giovanni.

I also mapped the space of the ER and its flux of people and resources by using in-site drawing as an ethnographic method. Through this set of tools, I developed the detail-oriented narrative style of the book. My hope is to do justice to the brisk, restless place that is the ER and to capture the immediacy of interactions and dynamics of attention.

This work was physically and emotionally challenging. I shared with patients, caregivers, and ER staff much more than my ethnographic project. We discussed anxieties and fears that the ER puts into focus, and we attended to people's pain and suffering. I shared with both patients and heath care providers a profound sense of frailty and discomfort. The ER qualifies among the "haunted" places of the hospital, where the stories of people whose death had been tragic never actually leave the ward (Street 2018; Varley and Varma 2018). Such stories are constantly shared among ER staff, and they recur in the nightmares of relatives, health professionals, and the ethnographer.

One more methodological decision needs to be accounted for. In the book, I focus upon interactions in which some form of urgency, demanded by relatives or patients and/or assessed by professionals, is implicitly or openly contested by one or more of the actors involved in priority-making. I decided not to focus on the more spectacular ER cases of massive bleeding, heart attacks, or violent head trauma due to car crashes, which correspond to "red codes"—that is, the most pressing and unambiguous cases of urgency.

My decision to look at urgency without focusing on extremely urgent conditions is at once ethical, analytical, and narrative. It is an ethical choice because whenever the ER received red codes, I was not able to closely observe interactions or gather diverse perspectives from the participants. Patients were unconscious; they had open wounds; their hearts were being resuscitated; their blood was gushing. Relatives were sobbing or shouting in sorrow and despair. Health care workers were doing their jobs with speed and care. In such circumstances, I put down my notepad and got out of the way.

My decision to avoid the most critical scenarios in the ER is analytical in the sense that it is through contestations and situations that do not perfectly match the ER's urgency evaluation criteria that the limited capacity to materially shape urgency in the ward is revealed. Focusing on conflicts, I foreground tensions and paradoxes of priority-making. While doing so, I illustrate the far-reaching, productive effects of those conflicts, capable of negotiating urgency by more generous terms and changing the governing of care within and beyond the ER.

My decision to examine urgency without focusing on critical situations is, finally, a narrative choice, in the sense that I wanted to write about a dimension of life in the ER that is generally overlooked—certainly in popular depictions. These days, there are countless representations of the ER on television and in movies, where attention is mostly devoted to moments of crisis in which health care staff rush off in a frenzy to save lives (and also to exploring the personal and romantic relationships of the ER staff). Perhaps unsurprisingly, most ER health care providers told me that they cannot stand television shows or movies about the ER.

But apart from such melodramatic representations, in real life the ER is also a place visited by people suffering from chronic conditions on a recurrent basis. It is a place where social isolation, homelessness, and invisibility, not readily apparent in many other public spaces, become tangible and real. The ER is a place of waiting just as much as it is a place of urgency and crisis. It is a space of failure as much as it is a space of healing.

After a brief history of the ER and Italian health care (chapter 2), in the chapters that follow I first look at how attention is socially distributed on the ward in terms of clinical triage (chapter 3). Then in chapter 4 I examine how the making of urgency in the ER carves out an experience of time that is alternatively structured around attention to the rating of risks, the slow-pacing of waiting, or the immediate market-driven desire for medical care. In chapter 5, I consider how shifts in attention are tied to widespread precarity and neoliberal national policies. This is followed by a chapter on how care practices in the ER are increasingly structured by mistrust (chapter 6) and by potential violence (chapter 7).

Addressing the particular positioning of the ER as a thick space of conjunction between neoliberal state politics and people's increasing need for care and recognition, in chapter 8 I address directly how what happens in the ER illuminates the caging nature of the welfare state in Italy, as elsewhere, before and after the COVID-19 pandemic.

2 · A CATHEDRAL OF BIOMEDICINE

One cannot fully appreciate the dynamics of triage in Italy as urgency in practice without a tour around a late medieval town, like the one that hosted the large university hospital where my fieldwork was held. In the maze of crooked alleys and terracotta-colored buildings, the power to determine who lives and who dies, as the governing of care distribution among the population, has left historical landmarks of all sorts.

Taking the 7:32 A.M. train to move toward the university hospital to follow the nurses' morning shift in the ER, I crossed the heavy stonework of what remains of the medieval town defense gates. At its heart is a monastery and its church, built in the fourteenth century. Its neat tower bell of light-gray stones is crowned with white marble sculptures of saints with iron halos, looking down with mercy on people passing by. Lit by the beaming September sun—just above its triangular summit—the monastery of the Lazzaretto was where the first people with leprosy, then people smitten by the black plague, asked for help from Dominican and Benedictine monks.

In the Middle Ages, the Catholic Church established itself as the main reference power over the suffering of the body and the soul. Suffering is at the heart of the Catholic theology of salvation. One must suffer as an atonement for sins, as a penitence for confessed guilt, and, finally, as a way toward forgiveness (Herzfeld 2009). The power to give attention to suffering is for the church one way to distinguish between salvific atonement and deserved punishment. By recognizing someone as worthy of help and salvation, Catholic authorities create people as subjects, as legitimate members of the Christian community.

Such attention creates a distributive power that was clear to noble families of the Italian Renaissance. The increasing demographic concentration in cities like Florence, Bologna, Venice, and Milan led to the proliferation of hospital centers. In Florence—one hour by train from where I was headed—between the tenth and the fifteenth centuries, fifty-eight hospitals were built, with about one bed per forty inhabitants (Cosmacini 2016). Those centers acquired a new status and became the wealthiest institutions in the city. Some remained active from the thirteenth century until today, like Santa Maria Nuova in Florence with almost 300 beds. Further, from the Renaissance onward the names of saints on health care structures were seconded by noble family names—Medici, Sforza, Borgia, or Este. This marked the birth of hospitals as a civic concern rather than only a matter of religious mercy (Cosmacini 2016).

A new change of demographics and the emergence of the capitalist market set in motion another sociological concern: one concerning the need for workers to be kept healthy. A landmark of such a new state of interests appears while the train skirts the medieval city center—an old hospital structure from the latter half of the eighteenth century, following Italian unification in 1861. With eclectic features that abandoned religious symbols, the building façade mixes columns and classic appearances with iron blossoms.

Hospitals' names, however, were not changed. Saints of the Catholic Church and the family names of nobles remained in place and are a powerful legacy today. Like ancient local celebrities, they stand in for local networks of solidarity and religious communities, de facto overcoming the legitimacy of the central state. Even the squared concrete buildings designed by the fascist regime carry the same local hospital names (Cosmacini 2016).

During a period regarded as the Italian "economic miracle" of the 1950s and 1960s, health care facilities of all sorts multiplied—pharmacies, elderly care homes, large hospital structures. Heading northwest, the train passes by many of those buildings, named after women—Villa Chiara, Villa Giulia, or Villa Cristina, in the case of various elderly care homes—or after rivers, hills, and local saints tied to geography in the case of pharmacies. The alleys of the city center are also rich with health care–related structures. Most are connected to each other by market arrangements. For instance, general practitioners (GPs) and pharmacies are often located side by side. GPs will recommend that their patients buy prescribed medications from their neighboring pharmacies, who, in return, pay GPs rent for their offices.

While these structures all struggle to capture patients' attention as consumers in the growing health care market, to the Italian state the redistribution of medical attention is a powerful instrument of local and national governance. Many contemporary Italian hospital structures built in the 1970s and 1980s—one I could see at a distance when the train finally left the city outskirts—were inaugurated during political elections to support local claims of opposing Communist and Christian party candidates.

Particularly in northern Italy, in places like the Emilia-Romagna region, Tuscany, and especially Lombardy, hospitals are the backbone of the national welfare system. For this reason, they are nowadays instruments of legitimacy used by all sorts of political entrepreneurs. The first of these was Silvio Berlusconi, multiply elected prime minister between 1994 and 2011. He contributed to the construction of a colossal hospital structure in Milan, the San Raffaele. The scenographic hospital architecture mixes statues of angels, Greek and Roman philosophers, and a sixty-meter-high helicoidal structure representing a string of DNA, covered by a wide glass dome. The place where I was headed was far more modest, and unremarkable, than these glorious hospital structures of the Italian past and present.

The train stopped at a little country station, the destination of all the passengers on board. The station, painted red and white, is a boxy construction made of prefab stucco and wide iron beams. Its style mirrors the imposing hospital building, about 30 meters high, that overshadows the parking lot in front of it, already packed with cars at such an early hour. Like a gothic cathedral, the hospital towers over the agricultural fields and the wide streets that connect it to the city center some 15 kilometers away. Difficult to reach for people not owning a car and having to pay for transport by bus, cab, or train (unavailable at night), access to this 94,000-square-meter-wide health care structure, worth about €190 million, takes money, time, and planning.

The attention that people sought in the Middle Ages, as pilgrims to a monastery, is alive in such a building, full of stern officialdom and religious influences. Its massive concrete structure has four floors supported by a series of round white columns. The vertical columns extend the entire height of the building from the basement to the roof. They punctuate the wide hospital façade, crowned at the summit with a triangular, temple-like roof. Of course, the hospital is named after a Catholic saint and a local noble family.

I got off the train and became part of the flow of people rushing forward through the parking lot in order to get to the main entrance of the hospital. On my first visit, I expected people who entered to stream away in different directions, separating down one or another of the multiple hospital corridors: to visit family members in a ward, to go to a scheduled doctor's appointment, or perhaps to be admitted themselves. Instead, most people who arrived with me on the train turned and went straight down a flight of stairs next to the hospital's cafeteria. They were heading toward a wide square building with a red-and-white metal arcade that read "Pronto Soccorso," the emergency room (ER).[1]

THE ER

The ER where I conducted my fieldwork between 2017 and 2018 is situated in northern Italy, in the Emilia-Romagna region. The region extends across the southern slice of the plains of the Po Valley, rich in medium- and small-sized industrial complexes and nestled between the Apennines and the shallow, warm Adriatic Sea. The landscape gradually changes from coastal pine forests to vast corn, soy, and cereal fields in the alluvial plains at its center. Farmland gradually transitions to hilly vineyards affected by ground erosion to rocky and increasingly wild hills as one moves toward the mountains in the west. The region is famous for its civic tradition and dynamic grassroots political activism. Bologna is its regional capital, and the region includes famous cities including Parma to the north and Rimini on the coast, to the south. It lies close to Veneto (the region of Venice) and Tuscany (with Florence, Pisa, and Siena), with easy access, too, to Lombardy (and so Milan, Como, and Bergamo).

Emilia-Romagna is one of Italy's twenty regions—administrative entities that enjoy wide-ranging administrative independence. Since 1992, health care has been administered by regional governments. The regionalization of health care in Italy (*regionalizzazione*) was introduced only a few years after 1978, the year the Sistema Sanitario Nazionale (SSN; National Health Service [HSN]) was established. Before then, since the unification of Italy in 1861, health care had been administered by cities at a local level (Cosmacini 2016). Today, the national government sets specific health care outcomes and budget goals (Livelli Essenziali di Assistenza [LEA]) that regions must meet annually. The LEA also works as the basis for regional planning and future health care financing from the central state. This system provides broad discretion to the regions so that in effect the Italian National Health Service consists of twenty different systems. This has exacerbated the historical north–south divide between regions that are more and less economically developed (Maciocco 2019). It has also made it difficult for the central government to maintain the same levels of assistance throughout the national territory. As a result, there is intense internal mobility of people from Italy's disadvantaged regions looking for health care within more advantaged places like Emilia-Romagna (Greco 2019).

Regions are divided into provinces and local health units (*unità sanitarie locali*). Since 1992, a local health unit may refer either to a city area or—as was the case for the university hospital where I did my fieldwork—an entire province (*azienda ospedaliera*, i.e., hospital agency). The ER in which I conducted my fieldwork is one of the main emergency hubs in the Emilia-Romagna region. It receives between 40 and 110 patients every day with staff who work eight-to-twelve-hour shifts composed of two to four physicians and five to six nurses (depending on whether it is a daytime or a night shift). Difficult cases are often transferred to this ER from other hospitals by ambulance or helicopter to access the high-quality specialized care offered there. Individual patients also travel from far away to reach this particular ER. It was not uncommon for me to sit in the external waiting room and speak with people who had traveled hundreds of kilometers to reach the place because of its reputation for biomedical excellence. Some people who had no car and lived in locations poorly served by buses or trains walked for several hours to reach the hospital, which was situated on the exposed side of the road in the middle of the plains of the Po Valley. This was an area baked by fierce sun in summer and chilled by freezing fog in winter. Others drove to the hospital from the nearby Apennines along narrow, winding roads.

The hospital serves a provincial area of around 700,000 inhabitants and is one of the two main hospitals in the area. The two hospitals share a common public agency (Azienda Ospedaliera) that acts as the joint administrator. Many of the medical specialties are divided between the two. For instance, the hospital where I conducted fieldwork is designated as a trauma and internal medicine center and includes neurology, cardiology, urology, intensive care, and psychiatry wards, among others. Pediatrics, gynecology, and ophthalmology wards (among others) are located in the other hospital, which is generally regarded as a women's and children's hospital and is located in the city center.

The hospital in which I did my fieldwork is a universe unto itself. Its labyrinthine corridors are composed of a seemingly infinite series of gray doors and white signs suspended from the neon-bright ceiling, punctuated by administrative offices and help desks. It has science fiction–like artifacts: high-tech operating rooms where artificial intelligence minimizes invasive surgical incisions and square robotic carts without drivers that carry heavy iron trolleys full of dirty sheets, scrubs, and lab coats to the ground-floor laundry. But the hospital is also a "haunted" place, where the metallic taste of blood sometimes almost imperceptibly appears on one's palate, and the astringent scent of medicalized death occasionally wafts unbidden into one's nostrils. It is full of abandoned corners and secluded spaces where enterprising homeless people try to find shelter, where stressed-out medical interns find rare moments of peace, and where I frequently ensconced myself to jot down field notes.

The anthropologists Sjaak van der Geest and Kaja Finkler (2004) have noted that the hospital is a space in which the stratifications and paradoxes that structure social life become overtly visible.[2] I thought of that perceptive observation every time I stepped inside the entrance to the hospital's main hall. Small flyers published by national unions that depicted nurses with decisively folded arms, advocating for improved health care and wage raises, contrasted with posters for private medical practices, glossy advertisements urging patients to try different kinds of medications, and lawyers' appeals to hire them to sue health care professionals.

The striking contrast between the ideas conveyed by advertisements like these appearing side by side aptly captured the situation of the hospital, and the Italian health care system more generally, at the time of my fieldwork. Health care providers such as nurses and doctors uniformly lamented their increasingly precarious working conditions. Many providers under the age of forty were able to access only short-term contracts with limited welfare benefits or with no benefits at all. Long-term or lifelong contracts, the norm in Italy during the 1980s and early 1990s (Molé 2011), had become rare, as public health care fell prey to austerity measures and neoliberal reforms.

Patients, in turn, found it increasingly difficult to access public health care services. Waiting times became epically lengthy, and perfunctory medical examinations became the norm. People who could afford to do so began going to private practices. At the same time, a widespread malcontent toward public health care initiated a torrent of lawsuits that targeted hospital staff. In the midst of such upheaval, the Italian population was aging, and socioeconomic inequalities were rising (Maciocco 2019). Requests for health care skyrocketed due to the growing presence of chronic, noncommunicable diseases and the absence of a systematic welfare response. In this context, both the patients and health care providers I spoke with felt increasingly sidelined, invisible, and precarious.

HOW HEALTH CARE IS ORGANIZED IN ITALY

Hospital reform is the first important step toward a social security system to be realized over a longer time scale.

—Cosmacini 2016, 494

With these words in the late 1960s,[3] the Socialist minister of health, Luigi Mariotti, declared hospitals to be a cornerstone of a renewed social contract between the state and its citizens. From the end of the Second World War, Italians had grown used to overcrowded wards and disastrously organized hospitals that provided fee-for-service health care in connection with work-related health insurance (*mutue assicurative*).

The first legislation on health care organization in Italy is dated, not surprisingly, after the Industrial Revolution in 1806. But due to the division of territory among different kingdoms, it was only in 1888, after the Italian Unification of 1861, that hospital legislation was nationalized under a shared law called Crispi and Pagliani, named, respectively, after the prime minister and the minister of health. What the law stated, though, is essentially the absolute independence of hospital institutions, be they managed by the military, the state, or, as was the case for the majority, the Catholic Church (Ginsborg 2006). The system left a lot of leeway in terms of how local hospitals were organized as fully independent administrative bodies.

There was no such thing as an ER. There were reception desks (*banconi*) at which people were summarily assessed by nurses who were not specifically trained for assessing urgency and who had no official guidelines to follow. Nurses based their judgment on their clinical experience and on their immediate impression of a person's suffering. A nurse's task was basically to sort those presenting and to determine who should be sent to a particular ward within the hospital, where a person could subsequently be fully attended to by doctors and ward nurses.

The health reform announced by Mariotti had long been awaited in the Italy of the "economic boom" of the 1950s and 1960s, during which time the country's increasing wealth was vastly unequally distributed. National newspapers and the international press regularly featured stories and images of sick people's agony—pitifully waiting in long lines in front of nurses' reception desks, trying to gain access to a bed in a hospital ward.[4] Health Minister Mariotti declared that his intent with hospital reform was to start the long path toward the application of the rights expressed by article XXXII of the postwar Italian constitution of 1948. This article states that "the Republic safeguards health as a fundamental individual right in the collective interest, and guarantees health care free of charge to the destitute."[5]

The law of 12 February 1968 created a regulated twofold system of care access: the hospital and the *ambulatori* (where local GPs practiced medicine). The hospital was privileged: it became an object of desire for people in need, in which *professori* (professors) and medical luminaries resided and dispensed alluring promises of healing. The *ambulatori*, on the other hand, remained largely disregarded by state funding.

Mariotti's law reconfigured hospital organization and created the *pronto soccorso*, the emergency room (Cosmacini 2016: 494–495). The ER became a proper department and not only a "reception desk." It became a practically and symbolically charged venue whose job it was to deliver care to people with the intention of prioritizing according to perceived clinical urgency, not only to prevent loss of life but also to help keep social injustice and political turmoil at bay.

Like many post–World War II European countries, Italy in the 1960s had a relatively young and healthy population that suffered mainly from acute issues such as workplace and road accidents, obstetric emergencies, and viral or bacterial infections that needed short hospital stays. By the late 1970s, however, people's health was increasingly associated with chronic conditions, requiring recurrent medical interventions and long-term medical support (Horton 2005; Manderson and Smith-Morris 2010). The Italian health service, which lacked a centralized organizational structure and was mostly based on fee-for-service health care, could no longer cover the increasing costs of people's care (Cosmacini 2016, 515). The violent political turmoil of the 1970s (later named the "years of lead," *anni di piombo*,[6] referencing the numerous shootings and assassinations of that decade) resulted in substantial political reforms.[7] This included the establishment of the Italian National Public Health Service in 1978, granting universal health care coverage and organizing health services on a national and local basis.

Before 1978, a unified public health care system did not exist in Italy. Rather, a series of fee-for-service health care facilities such as hospitals or outpatient clinics were created after the Second World War (and then partially reorganized in 1968 with Mariotti's law). As independent administrative bodies, the senior administration of hospitals and outpatient clinics decided on appropriate charges to patients for medications, surgery and examinations, and the organization of services. With the creation of the SSN in 1978, control over prices and health care organization passed to the Italian state. Health care became a fundamental right of the individual, rather than a service that was only accessible to individuals who could pay.

The Italian National Health Service today is a public system entirely funded by taxation revenue. Since regionalization in 1992, the state administers wide-scale planning by distributing funds regionally, thereby supposedly adapting national goals to local needs (Comodo and Maciocco 2011, 67–68). Local health units (*unità sanitarie locali*) administer general practice offices, mental health centers, hospitals, and administrative offices, according to municipalities and provinces. Large university hospitals, like the one where I conducted fieldwork, have their own administrations that work in coordination with local health units. All hospital funding is directly allocated by the region on the basis of budgets submitted. However, as it was originally conceived, the national health system lacked an overall system of organization of emergency services. How emergency services were provided varied even within the same region and local area, organized and administered by individual hospitals and not supervised by regional authorities.

In the years following the establishment of the National Health Service in 1978, ER services were mostly provided by physicians who rotated in and out on monthly shifts. Only nurses were specifically assigned to particular ERs. Recalling the 1980s, nurses and physicians told me that they worked all day and studied at night to reinvent their work from scratch. They read publications from UK and U.S. hospitals, where emergency medicine had already become an established field by the late 1960s (1967 in the United Kingdom and the year after that in the United States; Zink 2005). The late 1980s and early 1990s were years of experimental fervor, in which the ER was transformed from being the hospital reception of old—through which people were admitted for practical attention in the inner wards—to a place of specialized competence where needs were both sorted and addressed before eventually some but not all patients were admitted into inner hospital wards.

In 1992, a presidential decree (of 27 March 1992) created the current Italian emergency telephone number, "118."[8] Also in the 1990s, physicians started to be specifically assigned to the emergency ward as their place of employment, not simply as a place where they did monthly shifts. Professional associations started to appear, and in 2012, emergency medicine (*medicina d'urgenza ed emergenza*) became a national medical specialty with university training (Cosmacini 2016).[9]

But as the ER was changing, so, too, was the Italian NHS. The neoliberalization of Italian health care began in earnest in 1992 with government decree 502 (Cosmacini 2016). This decree started a process of *aziendalizzazione*, which meant that public health care facilities were to be managed much like private enterprises and had to follow new public management governance (Molé 2011; Muehlebach 2012).

Regions, local health units, and large hospitals became *aziende*—they became "public enterprises" rather than public health units (*unità sanitarie locali*). They became responsible for managing people's health care in ways designed to keep costs under control (Comodo and Maciocco 2011). A profound reorganization based on austerity measures and "rationalization of expenditures" (*razionalizzazione della spesa*) resulted in dramatic funding cuts and created a void that was readily filled by an already flourishing private health care market. The measures were initially justified as a way of containing the skyrocketing numbers of health care requests connected to the rise in chronic conditions that required long-term support (Maciocco 2019). One result of cutting funding and redirecting care responsibility from the state to the individual was an increase of health inequities among Italians, both in terms of access to and continuity of health care (Costa et al. 2016). State responsibility as a universal health care system—by that time, only just over a decade old—was increasingly withdrawn in favor of individual accountability, following the well-known neoliberal formulation of "no rights without responsibilities" (Pizza and Ravenda 2016).

The neoliberal reforms that reorganized the Italian health care system were part of a larger wave of political and economic reform. In Italy such reforms are associated with the repeatedly elected prime minister, Silvio Berlusconi, whose political reign lasted for almost twenty years (1994–2011). During those years, the Italian job market and social security system were transformed from a stable Fordist system, based on jobs for life, to a flexible model inspired by the English and U.S. job markets, premised on precarious working contracts (Tarì and Vanni 2005; Molé 2011).

As these reforms were being enacted, the Italian population was aging. Whereas in 1992 only 16 percent of Italians were aged sixty-five or above, in 2017 that percentage climbed up to 23.5 percent, making Italians the most elderly population of Europe, second only to Japan worldwide (Maciocco 2019). This meant a high prevalence of chronic noncommunicable conditions that required long-term support (40% of the Italian population in 2017 had at least one diagnosed chronic condition; Maciocco 2019). At the same time, the percentage of people living under worsening economic conditions increased. In 2017, more than 5.5 million people in Italy lived in "conditions of absolute deprivation," according to the National Institute of Statistics (ISTAT).[10] Unemployment had increased, too, especially among young people, and in 2017, 21.2 percent of people between fifteen and thirty-four were unemployed.[11] At the same time, Italy had also become a key transit destination for non-European migrants who since 2002, due to a series of increasingly draconian migration policies, had been cut off from accessing primary health care in Italy (Riccio 2007, 17–36; 2019; see Fassin 2011b).

These developments all impacted heavily on Italian health care generally and on ERs more specifically. As health care resources dwindled and as precarity swelled,[12] people increasingly attempted to cope in part with the precarity of their work, social abandonment, aging, and chronicity by coming to the ER to try to obtain medication, care, and attention.

Attention in the ER was demanded by patients trying to make themselves visible and was distributed by triage nurses. In the interplay between these two vectors, bodies became clinical objects (e.g., risks were defined, symptoms and palliation assessed, vital parameters taken), and people with complex social histories became absorbed as patients, subjected to the vicissitudes of factors such as the availability of stretchers and the length of the waiting list.

3 · TRIAGE AND ECONOMIES OF ATTENTION

Il triage è un porto di mare, una gabbia di matti!
Dove tutti entrano ma nessuno sa quando ne verrà fuori.
(Triage is a traffic port at sea. It's a madhouse!
Everybody gets in but nobody knows when they will get out.)
—ER nurse's remark on a busy Monday afternoon

Who decides when an urgent request for care is legitimate? How is such a decision made? The ER is a space where this question is negotiated daily. The ER is a place where different ways of understanding and handling bodies occur as a complex tangle of codes and numbers, fluids and masses, needs and suffering.

When a person arrives at the ER, they are assessed in terms of how urgently they need medical assistance. As I discussed in chapter 1, this assessment is called triage, from the French verb "to choose." The clinical triage evaluation process is intended to sort out people's medical needs and to see to it that they are attended by appropriate practitioners with access to appropriate resources. It constitutes the gateway of the emergency service. It is where priority is first allocated, needs assessed, and legitimacy bestowed. It is carried out according to fixed criteria, such as the evaluation of vital signs, state of consciousness, and clinical risk, and it is aided by material instruments such as checklists, charts, and various technologies that mediate between the health care provider's perception and the patient's body. But while triage is carried out with reference to fixed criteria, it is not done mechanically. Despite how it is described in medical literature, triage is highly dynamic. It is improvised and tailored to available resources and in relation to a wide range of other people's needs on the ward.

As I described in chapter 1, triage is the first of a two-step process by which urgency is governed in the ER. Those two steps are composed of initial clinical triage, then a doctor's examination. Clinical triage is carried out by nurses, who assign priority according to four color codes that have specific consequences for patients so labeled. These consequences are both temporal (less urgent codes mean longer waits) and financial (less urgent codes require the patient to pay more).

The lowest, least urgent code a patient can be assigned by a triage nurse is white. A white code means *utente improprio* (inappropriate user), indicating that the person really has no business in the ER: they may not be recognized to be sick at all by the triage team, or they should be going to their general practitioner (GP) for a consultation instead of taking up time and resources at the ER. The waiting time to see a doctor for a patient assigned a white code ranges between six and fourteen hours. It also incurs a €25 out-of-pocket "contact fee" and a co-payment (*compartecipazione alla spesa sanitaria*), a partial payment for the medical treatment, plus €23 more for each specialist examination or test done during the patient's time at the ER (the total sum is called *il ticket* in Italian).[1]

A green code indicates that the case is seen as either low urgency or nonurgent and might be assigned to a patient whom the nurse considers an inappropriate user. People assigned a green code usually wait from three to twelve hours to see a doctor. They will also have to pay the "ticket" fee if following their consultation, it is concluded that they were "inappropriate."

Yellow codes are urgent cases. They are high-priority codes. Waiting time ranges from twenty minutes to two hours. The only fees that such patients may have to pay are co-payments (fixed amounts paid by the patient for a particular service, from €23 to €36.15), depending on the type of specialist consultation and tests requested.

Red codes are unambiguous and treated as top priority: heart attacks, strokes, car accidents, shootings, stabbings, and so on. Red codes receive immediate attention and no fees are paid.

Codes are assigned as a result of the clinical triage assessment. One of the two triage nurses on shift writes their decision in the patient's records in the hospital's internal computer system. From then on, doctors and nurses inside the ward can check that system and see the code that a given patient was assigned. The nurse then communicates the color code to the patient, explaining the decision and the implications of the color code assigned. Communication is facilitated by an illustrated brochure (in Italian, French, Spanish, English, or Arabic) handed to the patient, with an *X* to mark the assigned color code. The brochure provides a standard explanation of what the color codes imply. It explains that a green code may be something like a sprained muscle, whereas a red code may be an acute heart attack. Even though this communication process may seem clear, most people I spoke with seemed to have no idea which code they had been assigned and why or what this implied in terms of waiting time and fee payment.

As in many Western European countries, Italy's national health system should in principle provide universal health care coverage to every citizen.[2] The *tessera sanitaria* (health care card) is a card issued to every Italian citizen attesting their right to be cared for in the national health service (as the Italian system is financed by taxation). It is issued by the regional authority, as health care in Italy is mainly region based. It is immediately requested in the ER as the scan reader automatically fills in patient data from the card. This digital system only works for people formally resident in the province (staff just need to know the name and surname as people are already in the database). The data on the card for people who are not residents is entered manually. Care is not denied to someone who has forgotten the card or does not have one since Italy has universal health care coverage; they are simply registered manually in the database.

In practice, however, the co-payment system (introduced in 2001) and the contact fees (introduced in 2011) were explicitly intended to curb the "misuse" of the ER. In the Emilia-Romagna region where I conducted fieldwork, there are exemptions from payment for people with a low income, migrants without a fixed address (*straniero temporaneamente presente*), and people with specific disabilities. These exemptions are not easy to come by. The low-income threshold applies to a very restricted number of impoverished people.[3] Migrants need a specific declaration as "without an address," which can only be obtained from the office that administers public health care waiting lists (Centro Unico di Prenotazione). Disability exemptions are available only to individuals who are estimated to have a functional impairment of at least 66 percent as certified by state-registered doctors (National Social Security Service, or the Istituto Nazionale Previdenza Sociale [INPS]). Most commonly, such individuals are in advanced states of Alzheimer's disease or other dementia, multiple sclerosis, or significant paralysis. Out-of-pocket contact fees may still be applied to anyone who health care providers decide has misused ER services.

Training textbooks describe triage as "democracy in action"—a practice that ensures equity of treatment to everyone, to the best of the health care providers' capacity (Aacharya, Gastmans, and Denier 2011). In reality, triage works according to two conflicting principles of justice and ethics. The first is that everyone should have access to care. The second is the more managerial concern of having enough resources to deal with care requests. This principle involves restricting access, ensuring that the people who need medical treatment most urgently actually receive it (Lachenal, Lefève, and Nguyen 2014).

But triage is much more complex than even these two ethical principles. It is an intermingling of the knowledge and demands of several actors—laypeople, ER staff, technologies of care, the medical bureaucracy—each with different access to and views about the events and the resources involved. Triage is a dynamic and recurrent assessment of a person's condition, in which multiple decision-makers and sources of uncertainty contribute to create urgency.

Multiple forms of triage also intersect within the decision-making about urgency that unfolds in the ER. This kind of triage is influenced by what happens before people call an ambulance or get to the ER by their own steam (by car, train, bus, or foot). Patients often consult with family members, friends, colleagues, or other health care professionals (like their GP or doctors on call on weekends or during festivities when there is a public holiday). When an ambulance is called, the patient's situation is examined by a prehospital triage assessment lead by distance, first, by the nurse operator of the emergency-call system (118) and on-site, later, by the ambulance workers.

In turn, the ambulance crew (trained volunteers, emergency nurses, and/or physicians) decides to which hospital to escort the patient. This decision is taken according to which medical specialties are located in each hospital, the distance between the location of the patient and the designated hospital, and whether the patient's health conditions allow a delay in transfer if the most appropriate hospital is at a greater distance.

After traumatic injury due to a car accident, for instance, the ambulance would bring those who are wounded to the hospital where I did my fieldwork, as a specialized trauma center. But if the car accident happened quite close to the city center and a person's eyes have turned reddish—as a result of copious internal head bleeding—the ambulance crew may decide to stop by the other closer hospital (pediatrics and gynecology, among other specialties) to stabilize the patient's condition before continuing to the appropriate hospital.

Whether patients arrive to the ER by ambulance or by their own means, key to understanding the multiple sources of uncertainty that create triage in practice is how the health care providers' attention is distributed. Attention in the ER concerns more than a psychological or a phenomenological capacity. Attention is a structuring feature that creates urgency. Its uneven distribution manages relations between patients and ER staff. The way attention circulates in the ER shapes the "relation between the visible and the invisible" (Foucault 2004, xiii): which conditions of suffering will be addressed; which needs can be legitimately expressed; which things matter most when people suffer. Both health care providers and patients (and their families or companions) try to control the way urgency is set by attracting or managing the way attention circulates in the ER.

JUST ANOTHER PANIC MONDAY

I enter the ER through the swoosh of the automatic glass door, and I am immediately hit by a sharp smell of sweat and astringent cleaning products. Yellow LED lights glow sharply against the institutional pale green flanks of the external waiting room. Chatter, coughs, and sneezing escort the sound of my steps. Directly across from the entrance, on the other side of the wide room that contains eighty blue plastic seats, there is a thick glass barrier surrounding the reception desk and the entire opposite wall. Information graphs and flowcharts hang near the entrance, providing explanations to visitors of what to expect from the ER. Colorful drawings of cartoon ambulances and hospitals made by local

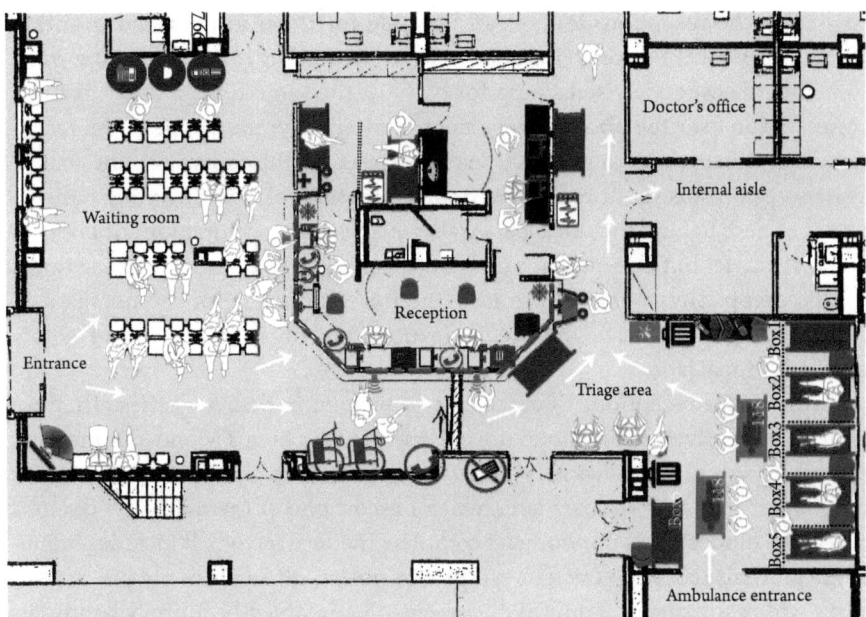

FIGURE 1. Map of the ER sketched by the author

elementary school children adorn the right side of the room, sprinkling its functional sterility with a few blooms of life.

People are uncomfortably seated on the stiff plastic chairs; a few lie across several seats. Some sit silently, suffering; others eat, chat, or sleep. Some people shout; others sit hunched over their mobile phones, texting. The television—a flat wide black screen—hangs in the upper-right corner near the entrance; a local commercial for a popular brand of sore throat pills is playing quietly as a backdrop to people's worries. Everyone in the room is waiting for something: loved ones, a doctor, another test, a hospital bed. A nurse who works in the ER once told me, "The emergency ward is one of the most important public places of the city." Surveying the range of people strewn about in the ER waiting room, I see what he means (see Figure 1).

Standing near the entrance and looking around, I note a woman and a man whispering anxiously to each other in an Eastern European language. The woman is holding her belly through her summer clothes. She sits chewing on her lower lip. An intravenous access inserted in her left arm is held in place by a couple of white bandages. The printed tag on the vial states "Libifen" in blue capital letters, a painkiller that is slowly dripping into her vein. Her baby son lies in a stroller, which she rocks back and forth to distract him. A man in his forties with intense brown eyes and a blue jacket holds her hand tightly while he stares at the glass barrier of the reception desk, clearly hoping for them to be called. Another woman's cry breaks through the chattering in the waiting room. Inside the ward, someone is desperately screaming for help. At the same time, a man sobs in a conversation over the phone; a boy laughs hysterically; the phone at the reception desk will not stop ringing. A tinny loudspeaker announces a patient's name. The receptionist is shouting, trying to make herself heard to incoming patients from her desk behind the thick glass wall, which effectively functions not only as a spatial barrier but also, perhaps unintentionally, as a sonic barrier. In the midst of this cacophony, everyone can hear the furious clacking of the nurse's keyboard typing—dull castanets clicking syncopated time like a burst of wildly improvisational jazz.

Close to the receptionist's office sit two women in their seventies. They are wearing expensive-looking floral dresses and are watching TV and commenting disapprovingly on the news they watch being broadcast. One is clutching a thick ring binder. As I will discover later, when I escort one of them into the doctor's office, the binder holds the woman's complete medical history. It includes homemade journals that keep track of symptoms, peeled-off labels of old pill bottles, and a wide assortment of official documents. It contains a beautifully handwritten index, sorted by year and type of document. This kind of careful documentation is not uncommon among chronic or elderly patients. Health care providers refer to documents like this caustically, dismissing them as the patient's "Holy Bible" (la loro Bibbia).

Patients' "Holy Bibles" were valuable instruments to triage nurses to orient themselves in the jungle of medical documents, though they were cautiously and at times suspiciously handled. People and their relatives' capacity to put order to professionals' examinations showed their in-depth understanding and firsthand long experience with the health care service.

To my left, along the aisle of seats, I see what seems to be a father taking care of his adolescent son, holding a pack of dry ice on his injured leg. The boy struggles to hold back the tears that seep out onto his Juventus club T-shirt. He sits in a wheelchair with his right leg lifted up by a shiny metal bar. Also clearly waiting for the orthopedic surgeon, two young women in their early twenties sit compulsively taking selfies, performing a "sexy-worried" expression (pouting lips, upturned eyes) to inform their social media friends that they are wearing neck braces due to a minor car accident. Meanwhile, a man who seems to be in his eighties, dressed in a flannel shirt and polished black shoes, a few white strands of hair carefully combed across his crown, waits his turn alone with shaking hands and a somber expression. A single tear slips down his lined face.

In gray work coveralls, two young African men wait for some news about their co-worker. Beside them sit a disheveled old man and a younger, elegantly dressed woman, who perhaps is his daughter. They lean toward an elderly lady with thick glasses to complain. "It's shameful that we've been waiting so long!

We pay taxes! It's all the immigrants' fault; they are not even waiting! They are always here for nothing! They are not even Italian!" the man exclaims, loudly enough for the African men to hear.

At the end of that same aisle of seats, I observe a skinny middle-aged man scrutinizing the instructions of a vending machine in order to figure out how to get an espresso. In the same corner of the room, a destitute-looking man, maybe homeless, tries to sleep despite the constant noise. His legs are thrust outward in front of him, and he has wrapped himself in a scruffy denim jacket. His shoes are almost completely worn out. He smells acrid and raw. Even though the waiting room is crowded, he is given wide berth.

The glass barrier opposite the main entrance where I am standing is punctured by three little round speaking holes and an opaque sliding door on the right side that allows people to enter and exit. The door is the focus of everyone's attention and worries. Beyond the door lies the place where triage is carried out. The majority of people wait, after having received a color code, to be called by nurses to finally access the doctor's office. The door thus serves as a portal to different hospital functions. It divides the external waiting room from the internal areas of the emergency ward. A small crowd of people continually collects there to try to attract the attention of ER staff.

A great deal of health care providers' work involves managing people positioned in front of the glass barrier or in the ER's internal area where triage is carried out. The health care providers grant some privacy to people who suffer greatly; they place dangerous or restless patients under their watch by keeping them in a visible isolated spot near the glass barrier; they try to manage relatives' anxiety by placing them far from where catheter changes, wound assessments, or other medical procedures involving blood and pain take place; and they prevent the formation of groups of onlookers that might obstruct ER staff activities.

The glass barrier ensures that patients cross its threshold by invitation only. Once they are called, they are allowed to pass through the barrier via the opaque sliding door. People stare at the glass wall, anxious and mesmerized, waiting to be called inside the ward to be examined by a doctor or hoping to see their loved ones reappear from the inside. The glass seems a live component of this border-land environment. It is like a display case; so much so that ER staff often call it "the aquarium." They say they feel like fish in a tank, while patients and the people who accompany them stand outside and scrutinize them.

The glass barrier is a sort of alert system for ER staff. It is a measure of people's anxiety. The longer and the closer people stand by the glass, the more they want to get in to be attended to by health care providers. Some people behave like geckos, pressing their hands on the glass, eagerly looking inside, attentively scanning movements, looking for any trace of change within the inner ward. They assert their presence with their intent, focused gaze. This rarely helps. Whenever anyone asks when it is going to be their turn, they are usually sent away with "No time estimate possible; there are still a few patients ahead of you." Patients do not have access to the waiting list—the digital display that had been promised to ER staff some months prior has so far not materialized. When they ask, patients are only given a rough estimate of the number of people who need to access care before them; they are also reminded that the number can change at any minute should people with more urgent medical needs suddenly arrive.

As I move close to the glass barrier, the emergency signal on the top of the opaque sliding door suddenly lights up. A well-dressed couple in their forties storm into the waiting room and start questioning the receptionist, panting heavily. They are the relatives of a red-code patient who just arrived by helicopter. They insist on knowing further developments. "There are none for now, but that's good," says the receptionist, always a sociomedical aid worker, not a nurse, reassuring them from behind the glass.[4]

Behind the glass barrier, two triage nurses sit beside the receptionist. Although they wear scrubs instead of a blue uniform like the receptionist, patients do not distinguish among them. A triage shift is composed of two nurses wearing full white scrubs with marine blue neckbands;[5] a staff badge pinned to their chests, sometimes with a stethoscope around their necks; and always an arsenal of pens, scissors, and bandages protruding from their pockets.

Nurses constantly struggle to manage the continuous flow of requests from people who come to the ER as patients, as external professionals (e.g., police, firefighters, ambulance staff), and as personnel from various hospital wards. Someone asks for information: "Sorry, where is the urology department? Can I pass through here to go there?" Others ask if they can go inside to visit a relative or a friend in the inner waiting room or in the intensive observation unit, Osservazione Breve Intensiva. The question "How long will it take to call me? Where am I on the patient list?" recurs incessantly. Meanwhile, the emergency phone does not stop ringing, providing information on incoming cases, demanding updates on old ones, looking for professionals on duty, asking about available beds for patients waiting to be admitted, looking for blood supplies or medications, and asking about bureaucratic processes.

Behind the glass wall, one of the two triage nurses who sit next to the receptionist is totally absorbed in her typing. I pass by her, making a quick gesture to say hello. She responds with a rapid smile while she continues to glance at the computer screen, the people in front of her on the other side of the barrier, and the ringing phone. I open the door in the left-inner corner of the waiting room, at the rear of the reception desk, and enter the "advanced triage" office. I close the glass door behind me. Suddenly, the world turns relatively silent. I exhale. This private room of opaque walls is used by nurses to let off steam during chaotic overcrowded shifts. People who need a private, less hectic environment during their wait are placed on the two stretchers pushed against the walls of the room. A white curtain cuts it in half.

I get my lab coat from the inner office of the head nurse. I take my recorder and notepad out of my backpack and leave the backpack behind in the head nurse's office with my sweater and raincoat.

One last breath and I am ready to dive in, shadowing nurses doing triage.

MAKING URGENCY BY CONTROLLING ATTENTION

On average, every eight seconds we get interrupted by something.

—Young ER doctor

In the overcrowded ER, attention is a scarce resource. Drawing on the sociologist Pierre Bourdieu's (1977) practice theory, attention here can be seen as a kind of capital, something that by its nature is finite and hence can only be maintained or obtained at something or someone else's expense. For this reason, I will speak of an "economy of attention." The term has widely been used by media scholars to describe the commodification of attention by social media platforms.[6] Here I use "economy of attention" differently. I engage triage as an example of what can be practically "done with" attention, other than attention being considered a property (a having) or a state of mind (a being; Citton 2017). I retain the metaphor of an "economy of attention" to illustrate the creation of difference, a trade-off between what is made visible and what is kept waiting within triage interactions in the ER.

As a resource, attention is relational: it is "paid to" and "received from." In a circular movement, the giving of attention creates value, and what has value attracts people's attention (Derber 2000). To identify the ways in which attention works is a "powerful instrument for understanding how people respond to, interpret, and engage with their surrounding world" (Throop and Duranti 2015, 1057).

Like all economies, attention is vulnerable to change. The philosopher Edmund Husserl explains that attention is "affected" by the "pulls" of the surrounding world (1962, 27–92). In the ER, the capacity of both incoming patients and health care providers to pay attention and receive it is determined by their different degrees of socialization within the ER environment and by their relative authority and power within the setting. But attention is also subject to sources of uncertainty and new events—for example, the arrival of an ambulance or the rapid deterioration of a patient's condition. Events like these "forcefully steer attention from the outside" and thereby redefine what is attended to first (Schroer 2019, 425–426). Nurses on the front line of triage assessments have to learn ways of trying to control the economy of attention that enables their work.

Coding situations and prioritizing relations are taught to nurses first during the obligatory national training course given by the Triage Training Group (Gruppo Formazione Triage [GFT]) and second by their initial ward-based training shadowing an expert nurse for an average of two weeks.

Following official guidelines and class training, triage has a four-step outline:

(1) On the spot evaluation
(2) Short structured interview (also called subjective data collection [*raccolta dati soggettivi*] or anamnesis)
(3) Patient examination (objective data collection [*raccolta dati oggettivi*])
(4) Possible reevaluation (not mandatory; depends on available time and developments in the patient's condition)

The first three of these steps take from three to fifteen minutes to complete; the fourth is optional. These steps frame nurses' practical efforts to control the way their attention is distributed in the ward by prioritizing relations—that is, *mettere le cose in fila* (literally, "to put things in line"), thereby letting urgency come into being. But local practice is more fluid than class training or official guidelines. Different steps of triage are skipped, merged, repeated, and recontextualized according to resources at hand, habits, and other necessities.

FIRST STEP: "BAD" AT FIRST SIGHT

You can really tell what they have as soon as they walk through the door. The way they look, talk, walk, and gesture gives you all that you need.

—Emergency doctor, during a quiet early morning

"I don't like this; he looks bad" (*è brutto*). This expression, *brutto* (literally, "ugly"), is frequently used by triage nurses when they are confronted with a patient who seems seriously ill. The expression refers to the nurses' sense that a patient "doesn't look right" (*ha una brutta cera* or *faccia*) and that what is affecting them might need urgent attention. In ward jargon, this quick on-the-spot judgment constitutes the first step of triage, called "first look" (*colpo d'occhio*, literally, "eye shot"). It is how nurses immediately sense danger, matching patients' appearance with possible medical danger. The anthropologist Andrew McDowell, looking at general practice in India in the context of global health interventions, referred to such kinds of "intuition" within triage as its "ordinary affects," the ways in which triage is "inhabited and animated" by "not-reflexive" ways of spotting and making a difference (2019, 306).

The first look enacts a field of visibility where hidden issues are sought out. This aesthetic judgment is not limited to signs shown by people's bodies (e.g., bleeding or visible swelling; appearing reddish, pale, or yellowish; limping or shaking, etc.). Beyond clinical guidelines, nurses learn to notice details such as clothes, smells, and attitudes, which reveal something about the working conditions, pain endurance, severity of suffering, habits, and chronic conditions that affect the patient—thus focusing the health care providers' minds on certain possible risks. The first look mainly unfolds in front of the glass barrier if patients arrive at the ward on foot or in the internal waiting room if they have been brought to the ER by an ambulance or some other vehicle.[7]

A person's face (referred to by ER staff by the Latin medical term *visus*) has particular importance in how triage nurses evaluate them. People who look "reddish" (*rossore*) might be suffering from hypertension. Being pale can be read as anemia or internal/external bleeding. Yellowish can mean liver problems; gray can signal an imminent heart attack. "Cherry-like" (*color ciliegia*) can mean carbon monoxide poisoning.

The reading of the *visus* regards three basic features: skin color, body signs (sweat, drops, blood, scars, burns, hematomas, stains, paralysis, etc.), and emotional state. Bodily signs are also read. A patient who holds their lower abdomen might be indicating kidney stones; keeping their back slightly bent over—while walking or sitting—lower back pain, such as lumbago. Shaking can mean neurological problems or shock. Cramps can indicate that the patient is cold or extremely frightened. And so on.

Olfaction also plays a role in this first approach. An experienced triage nurse is able to smell the particularly acrid sweat of a patient with liver problems or hepatitis. The scent of ketones suggests an individual is in diabetic shock. The "smell of street" (*odore di strada*) reveals instead a desperate socioeconomic condition and lack of housing. The penetrating odor of gangrene, blood, feces, and urine and the scent of people's perfume, skin, clothes, and breath (alcohol, smoke, vomit, drugs) provide nurses with other embodied clues. Smell places a barrier around patients, hitting health care providers' noses with the invisible threatening presence of viruses and bacteria. Often, nurses wear protective masks, use many pairs of plastic gloves, and clean their hands twice using antibacterial gel, generally limiting contact with patients and handling their bodies as contagious by default. This was so even when I conducted my fieldwork before the COVID-19 pandemic; since then, they *always* wear protective respirators, as well as many other articles of protective clothing.[8]

The patients being read by the ER staff in return try to read the health care providers. Stereotypes play an important role in first sight exchange, redirecting urgency and attention. For instance, health care providers with a southern Italian accent are sometimes dismissed by patients as *sfaticati* (lazy), reflecting a long history of north–south prejudice and antagonism in Italy. Health care providers also often portray people coming from southern Italy, particularly from the Campania region around Naples, as exaggerating their suffering and being melodramatic. The same is often said about migrants from sub-Saharan Africa or the Maghreb.

Female health workers are also subject to stereotypes, particularly if they are young. Patients appeal to males—any male, including medical know-nothings like me—as *Dottore* (Doctor). Female health care providers, on the other hand, are often called Signorina, "Miss," even when they are doctors. Health care providers are sometimes not much more enlightened: women are less likely to be believed when they report suffering, especially when they are judged attractive. As the anthropologists Julie Livingston (2012) and Alice Street (2014) have pointed out in very different contexts, in the ER variables such as class, ethnicity, gender, and their multiple intersections do not disappear; instead, they entangle patients, ER staff, and their families in intricate sociopolitical hierarchies.

SECOND STEP: "TELL ME, WHAT IS GOING ON?"

They never make it easy! They always say things in the weirdest ways.
—Young nurse complaining about nurse-patient communication

The second step of triage is a structured interview called *collezione dei dati soggettivi* (subjective data gathering). The goal of this interview is to collect symptoms and the patient's story, following the question pattern SAMPLE, an acronym for "symptoms, allergies, medication, past illnesses, last oral intake, events leading up to the present situation."[9] This interview usually takes place in front of the glass barrier between the patient and the nurse, but it can also occur in the internal waiting room or in the more private setting of the "advanced triage" office. The space is sometimes changed during the course of the interview if, for instance, a patient needs to lie down, sit, or have privacy while they speak. To be granted some privacy and a stretcher in the inner area is a sought-after, valued asset in the overcrowded ER. Nurses remark tartly that "as soon as people enter the sliding doors, suddenly they lose their ability to walk."

In the ER, it is not always easy to talk, as a result of background noise, the general lack of privacy and time, possible language barriers, breathing or hearing difficulties (when the interview takes place through the glass wall), panic, anxiety, confusion, and the general lack of awareness of what to expect. Interruptions, hesitations, emphasis, and overlapping speech all occur as data for both patient and health care practitioner. The interview directly affects both the nurse's view about patient health and trustworthiness and the patient's trust in ER staff work.

A further complication concerns the person who speaks and how they speak. Patients are often accompanied by relatives, friends, and loved ones, who in many cases interrupt or attempt to complete patients' accounts. Sometimes, for example when patients are elderly or unconscious, caregivers or ambulance staff are the only ones who speak. The way people speak for the patient is telling for health care providers and can suggest tensions or conflicting views. When too many people speak for a patient and communication is getting out of hand, a strategy employed by many nurses is to ask, "Wait, who's the patient here?," demarcating first- and secondhand knowledge among interacting participants.

Nurses also pay attention to what is not said. When they are unsure about a patient's story, they sometimes try to recreate a "safe space" (*uno spazio sicuro*) by granting more privacy, usually in the advanced triage area, and to actively divert the patient's attention by talking about something else besides discomfort or pain (for example, "What do you do for a living?"). The intention behind this strategy is to separate the patient from obstreperous caregivers, to invite an emotional response, to actively engage with the patient's life, and, of course, to gather useful information. In a sense, triage nurses create a "confessor role" to try to sort out potential contrasts and conflicts among parties and better understand people's intentions.

To contextualize risk and confirm or confound patients' narratives, triage nurses look at medical record sheets brought in by patients (including their "Holy Bibles"), their medications (as a way to assess allergies and chronic conditions), and scars and signs of precedent distress and surgeries (during the third phase of signs evaluation). They also check the ER's digital intranet network to access previous medical examinations and diagnoses that may have occurred there in the past.

Managing Information

Triage interviews vary in terms of how successfully they achieve their goal of focusing the nurse's attention on health care priorities. Here are three short examples of how interactions may unfold during the second step of triage, which highlight some common ways for nurses to manage information provided by patients:

1. A gray-haired man in his late forties, still dressed in his blue work coverall stained with engine oil, reports a workplace accident that occurred an hour previously while he was assembling a car at a factory nearby. This happens frequently in the area near the hospital, called the Italian Motor Valley, headquarters of internationally famous brands such as Ferrari, Lamborghini, Maserati, and Ducati. The man has a strong Emilia-Romagna accent: the first syllable of words is stressed while the last is kept long and open, and "s" is uttered softly, as in the English "shock" or "share." The man's narrative is punctuated by the expression *du maròn* (literally, "two chestnuts" or "two balls"), which means that something is annoying. The man gives the nurse his health care card and tells me and the nurse that he strained the muscle of his left thigh and heard a sudden *ciocco*, a snap, while leaning over. It hurts badly. The nurse had noted him limping his way into the ER. She asks him to tell her where exactly it hurts and fills in the eform for work-related injury, the INPS declaration,[10] and charts a care path for the man, leading toward an X-ray and orthopedic examination. She assigns him a green code and gives him a painkiller while he waits to see a doctor.

2. The triage nurse interviews a well-dressed middle-aged woman who says she suffers from constant headaches and dizziness, without nausea or vomiting. She complains about her GP. She has come to the ER to seek a second opinion. The triage nurse recognizes the situation: many patients come to the ER because they are not happy with their GPs. Still, he wonders aloud why the woman has not changed her GP: it is so simple! He looks at the handwritten prescription from her GP, trying to understand the GP's illegible writing. He asks the woman if her headache has somehow changed recently.

"It's kind of a new thing," she replies. "It's like having ants going around in my head."

"Like a tingling?"

"No, like ants."

The triage nurse nods, unconvinced. He asks the woman if her dizziness feels like she is whirling in a steady environment or if she feels that the rest of the world is spinning around her. "A mix of both," she says.

The nurse turns around and shoots me an ironic, knowing look. He seems not to trust the woman's description. But her report of a "new thing" might still indicate something worthy of a green code.

3. The triage nurse addresses an elderly woman, saying "Hello, how may I help you?" She responds: "I fell down the stairs last Sunday. It seemed not to hurt that much so I wanted to take care of my back by myself with some ointments, but then last night I couldn't sleep for the pain, and then I got scared so I came here for a checkup."

"I'm sorry, Madame," the nurse says in an assertive tone. "This is an emergency ward; you had the accident a week ago. An emergency is something that happens immediately after the fact. Now you should go to your GP. We only deal with emergencies here. I will put you on the waiting list but you are a white code. I'm telling you: there's a long wait because if we get a real emergency, that will take precedence over you."

The first example, of the man who had suffered a workplace accident, was unproblematic for the nurse; she immediately perceived what needed to be done. It was a classic acute case that respected all emergency ward assessment criteria. The here, the now, the biological, and the objects of medical and legal concern were easily absorbed into ward infrastructures.

The second example differs from the first since the background request was a second medical opinion of a diagnosis that had already been given by her GP. The GP's prescription could not be read, which raised the issue of care fragmentation among different public services. The male nurse was sympathetic to the woman, but in his view she had an "unconcerning" (*non rilevante*) way of describing how she felt. It was difficult for the nurse to accept "a tingling sensation going around my head" (*un formicolio che gira nella testa*) as a reason to admit the woman to the ER system. In addition, the woman's definition of dizziness did not match clinical descriptions of vertigo. To turn the woman's subjective state into an objective medical sign, the nurse focused on the only relevant clue he could extract: "It's kind of a new thing." A person suffering from frequent headaches can recognize changes in experienced pain, marking an upcoming new event. Therefore, in this case the situation was defined as changing and at risk of developing further. A certain timing was given to the suffering, which was compatible with the clinical definition of urgency, as an emerging event. Her need was translated into a legitimate green code.

The opposite of all this is the third example. After dismissing the patient with a white code, the nurse turned to me and said, "If she has waited so long to come here, she can wait some more. It is certainly not serious." On this occasion, the woman ended up waiting more than six hours for the doctor to see her. If she had come to the ER right after her fall, she probably would have been classed as an acute case, like the first example. Another path would have been to go to her GP and then, eventually, come to the ER in case of no improvement. In the latter case, she would have been nonurgent but considered as low urgency, like the second example. Here though, the woman was identified by the nurse as a "line cutter" (saltare la fila), as someone who wanted to avoid the often substantial waiting time to see a GP in order to get a quick X-ray and intravenous painkillers (she later revealed to me that she did not have the time to go to her GP as his office hours did not match her work schedule).

In all three examples, the nurse's selection of relevant information was based on an idea of urgency rooted in a biomedical understanding of what it is like to have a break in normal functioning that requires immediate intervention after the first appearance of symptoms or after a worsening situation. Such understanding of urgency depicts an individual body as split between an inner dynamic that, if truly painful, cannot be ignored and a blurry external reality that has little relevance to health care providers' work. When people arriving at the ER turn from people into patients by the code allocated to them, they are expected to sacrifice part of their subjectivity and agency in order to become objects of medical knowledge and intervention.

On the other hand, the people who come to the ER understand pain and risk through their everyday lives. For them, urgency is often experienced as more than merely a biomedical event. As I illustrate in the following chapters, people's social relations, work, families, and loved ones also play an active role in defining which symptoms and changing behaviors might be understood as worrisome and which instead might not trigger appraisal and fear and thus do not escalate into a help-seeking scenario. As the anthropologist Ayo Wahlberg and colleagues argue in relation to diagnostic pathways for childhood cancer, the perceived urgency of a condition also depends on people's abilities to access medical or social aid (Wahlberg et al. 2020).

As the above examples indicate, a key role is played by people's relationships with their GPs. In chapter 5, I further explore these relationships that enable or deny people access to medical specialists and in-depth diagnostic examination and show how this has an important effect on ER overcrowding.

THIRD STEP: LOOKING FOR SIGNS

The third step of triage is called *raccolta dati oggettivi* (objective exam evaluation). This concerns the physical examination and evaluation of the patients' body and the monitoring of basic vital signs and is carried out either in the advanced triage area or in the internal waiting room. Measurements taken are heart rate, breathing/oxygen saturation, and blood pressure. Making an evaluation using the Glasgow Coma Scale, for state of consciousness, is added and—if needed—also temperature, electrocardiogram (ECG), and an evaluation using the Cincinnati Prehospital Stroke Scale (CPSS). These tests are done by approaching the patient with a set of mobile machines wheeled around the ward on stainless steel trolleys.

In this phase, patients' bodies are touched, their vital signs are observed, and their pain evaluated through questioning, using a numerical rating scale (NRS) from zero, "not painful at all," to ten, "worst pain imaginable" (or a VAS visual analog scale; Williamson and Hoggart 2005). The NRS scale is not really trusted by nurses, who remark: "Of course, if you ask people everyone is a ten or a nine, everybody says ten because nobody wants to sit in the waiting room." The application of NRS guidelines reveals more about health care professionals' views of patients' subjectivity than it does about pain experienced. It provides the ER staff with ideas about who is able to endure pain and who is not (Johannessen 2019).

In this phase, bodies are observed for hidden, invisible presences that could have an impact on their health. Through palpation and medical semiology—that is, the set of physical manipulations that constitute the bedside diagnostics that clinicians use to interpret signs in the body—these forces are actively brought to the fore. Signs are gathered in the search for probable causes and risk of further development. A dialogue with those forces is established by ER staff by sensing, probing, and palpating body parts while imagining obscure entities such as organ inflammation, vein swellings, blood stoppages, and fecalomas (blocks of feces stuck in the intestines).

It is not unusual to witness a nurse addressing a body part. An absorbed nurse will direct a needle at an arm, urging a vein: "Come on! Where are you? Don't tell me that you are empty! Don't you have even a drop of blood for me?" In a call and response game of tinkering, body parts and symptoms are handled carefully because they are never a straightforward presence. They might reveal themselves as misleading and change over time—like an apparently relaxed abdomen of a person feeling dizzy that hardens all of a sudden, turning tense and swollen due to undetected copious internal bleeding—or they might confound clinicians' ideas about relevant signs and symptoms.

This dialogue with bodily parts attempts to shape living matter in accordance with the technical processes in the ward. As diagnostic tools such as X-rays or computer imaging make organs, bones, and muscles visible, so nonhuman actants across the body are enacted, gathered, and brought to life through handling, probing, and palpating. As the philosopher Annemarie Mol (2002) has shown, in clinical work different ways of enacting disease coexist, crafted by several practical approaches to the body. Processes like the CPSS to determine stroke, abdominal palpation, or evaluations of consciousness bring organs and nerves into epistemological focus. They enact biology by rendering its objects present in the immediacy of the assessment. They turn people into assemblages of biological risks. As an example:

Beep, says the blood pressure machine standing on the trolley of the advanced triage area. *Beep*.

"Let me connect the cable again," says the triage nurse bending over to collect the link cable of the blood-pressure cuff. "Let's do this again. Could you please take off your sweater; it's kind of tight on your arm, so it might affect the result."

The middle-aged man, who came to the ER right from work and is still wearing paint-stained trousers and safety shoes, nods and takes off his sweater.

The nurse then slips the cuff onto his thick arm. "Okay, one last time."

Beep. She clicks start and the cuff begins to inflate. The machine seems to be working this time.

The numbers on the display climb up and down while the cuff deflates. They finally stabilize with a *beep*. The result is not that different from before. At 180/107 the numbers almost qualify the man to be given a yellow code.[11] But the experienced nurse is unsure what to do.

"Are you nervous?" she probes the patient.

"No, I am feeling fine."

"Do you usually have high blood pressure?"

"No, actually it's usually kind of low."

"Mmmh," nods the nurse.

The man has not been taking any hypertension-related medication either.

"Stay here so you can calm down a bit, and we'll try again in ten minutes."

Two different versions of this situation are outlined: the automated blood pressure cuff indicates dangerous hypertension, while the patient says he is calm. The nurse has to decide what to do. She lets the patient rest for some time (she is still convinced that he is scared and nervous) and tries to measure his blood pressure again. This time, she takes his blood pressure manually, sensing the pulse with two fingers and listening to his heartbeat with a stethoscope as the sphygmomanometer inflates and deflates.

Trusting their own capacity to hear and judge, the majority of the staff in the ER think that manual methods are generally more accurate than machine-generated ones. The hands-on manual way of taking blood pressure, for example, is not liable to faulty cable connections, signal troubles, or the freakish behavior of lithium batteries. In this case, the man's blood pressure had gone down. The nurse read this change as confirming her hypothesis of what is called the "hospital effect" (*l'effetto ospedale*)[12]—that is, the fear people feel when they go to the ER, when not knowing what will happen is reflected in elevated blood pressure.

This explanation served the triage nurse's interest in delaying the man's entrance to the ER, assigning him a green code instead of an urgent yellow one in order to let another of "her" patients into the doctor's office: a frail elderly woman next in line on the green-code list.

Pacing the admittance of patients is a common practice, particularly during busy days and during shifts staffed by new or inexperienced doctors, who are slower in completing examinations. A major concern of triage nurses is the gap between the low-urgency green codes and the priority yellow ones. They have introduced a "yellow B" code in order to deal with borderline cases that are less serious than yellow codes but cannot afford to wait as long as green codes. This borderline code has multiple uses according to the situation at hand. It can be used to prioritize particularly frail elderly people, to favor a distressed child, to push forward a case that is unclear to the nurse, or to assist someone who is suffering greatly.

In the third step of triage, nurses feel that they can access "the stuff" (*che succede*, literally, "what happens"), the cause of distress, through direct contact—seeing, touching, and measuring what is going on—rather than relying on accounts from patients and caregivers.

In reality, things rarely work out that way. Diagnostic machines foster peculiar ways of engaging with people's bodies, and they do not simply reveal what is already "there" as an object to be discovered. Rather, by attending to what they are able to capture, nurses and patients "mediate" their perception and sense-making (Latour 2007, 33). Diagnostic machines are not neutral, and as nurses are well aware, results need to be contextualized in the current situation, which in turn validates or disclaims the work of diagnostic machines. By interpreting test results, professionals translate diagnostic measures into practical action. They do this mainly by relying on their experience in "sensing danger," in dealing with the corporeality of the suffering body, and in navigating situations by seeing, touching, smelling, and hearing that something bad might be going on.

Wrapping Things Up

When the third phase of evaluation has been completed,[13] the triage nurse needs to decide upon the color code. At this point, the nurse usually retires to their computer to sort out their impression of the situation, what they have noted through examination, the patient's report of previous medication, and, usually, a pile of medical records brought in by patients or the ambulance staff and spread out on the desk. Nurses flip through the papers scattered around the table next to their monitor, separating them out from other people's records and hospital forms. If the patient has handed the nurse a plastic bag full of the medications that they have been taking recently (as often happens), the nurse will rummage through that. The nurse then makes a list of the most relevant medications—antidepressants, anticoagulants, blood pressure medications, painkillers, antibiotics, insulin, and so on. Meanwhile, they try to figure out how to represent the situation within the few lines of triage notes, justifying their choice of color code based on available data. The nurse starts with the usual medicolegal frame: vigilant, eupneic (i.e., normal breathing), conscious, oriented, compliant patient . . .

The nurse then describes events and symptoms, followed by an account of their current medical evaluation and notes about the patient's past chronic conditions, diagnostic evaluations, and a list of relevant allergies and medications. Writing things down allows the nurse to sort the present and past history of people, signaling available options for intervention.

Nurses seek to manage the inflow of patients to the ER without jeopardizing the economy of attention that supports their work. When this is not possible, they try to fast-track the patient's entrance into the ER doctor's office, called *sponsorizzare* in ward jargon, or redirect them to specialists in other wards; the latter option is available only in limited cases according to specific hospital protocols.

Triage notes are also produced in awareness of the ever-present threat of litigation, as I discuss in chapter 4. In addition to providing crucial medical information, the notes are also considered to be written "for the judge," following the accountability principle: "If you haven't written it down, it did not happen and you have not done it." To avoid accusations, nurses follow a reversal principle: the lower the code, the more probable contestations and problems with patients, so the more precise triage notes and risk evaluation need to be. The same goes for situations in which other state institutions are involved; for example, collecting proof related to criminal charges (*trattamento sanitario obligatorio*), forced psychiatric treatment, or the care of prison inmates.

FOURTH STEP: REEVALUATION

The fourth step of triage, reevaluation, occurs only if there is sufficient time. It takes many forms, according to different situations, spanning from a simple reassuring "How are you feeling now?" to a complete rechecking of basic vitals or a second ECG and other instrumental tests. Reevaluation has a managerial role: giving attention is a way of managing the "mood" of the waiting area, defusing tension, and preventing violence, particularly during busy shifts and resource shortages. After the procedure, the color code assigned may change to represent potential escalations (e.g., green codes may develop into yellow or, more rarely, into red ones).

ATTENTION AS A DRIVING FORCE AMID TRIAGE

As should be clear from this description of the four steps of triage, urgency is intersubjectively driven and enacted as a way to attend, objectify, and manage matters that demand attention. Relations emerge as relevant by directing health care providers' attention to the task of crafting objects of knowledge. The creation of urgency and its coding depends on the possibility of "infrastructuration": the possibility of being able to connect patients' issues with resources in the ward, visibility, and validation through attending, defining, and circumscribing the issues and appearances deemed relevant by triage staff (Larkin 2013). Attention creates the links that constitute the daily infrastructure of the ER, and its circulation is key to infrastructuration. Work flows and gridlocks are both linked to the work and circuits of attention, which may be responsible for swift changes in, or the falling apart of, assemblages of people, bodies, spaces, and technologies.

Attention is the most desired resource inside the ER. People constantly try to grab health care providers' attention, while nurses do their best to avoid looks coming from outside as they focus on the subtle signs of pain and disease and their immediate tasks at hand. Attention is a matter of visibility and positioning, of turning toward certain actors instead of just glancing over them (Csordas 1993, 138). Attention is mobilized through bodies and actions that shape intersubjective processes (Csordas 1990, 1993; pace Merleau-Ponty 2013).

In her research in a hospital in Papua New Guinea, the anthropologist Alice Street (2014) reverses Foucault's (2003) analysis of the hospital as a panopticon where people are constantly observed and controlled. In the hospital where she worked, "doctors sense their marginality to global science and its publishing networks. . . . Nurses become aware of their own irrelevance to managers, politicians and bureaucrats," and "patients come to see themselves as peripheral in relation to a world of white people's knowledge and expertise" (Street 2014, 232). She describes the hospital she worked in as a place where people struggle to be seen, where needs fail to be engaged, and where invisibility is a sign of state failure.

Although it is far from Papua New Guinea, it seems possible to find a parallel with the ER in Emilia-Romagna. People as subjects in the ER engage in an "everyday struggle to mobilize techniques of visibility" (Street 2014, 232). To avoid fading into the background of the "generically sick" and to navigate simultaneous events (Street 2014, 226), patients in the ER where I worked strategically positioned themselves in passageways in order to be noticed; health care providers tactically pretended not to hear people yelling to get attention, and they avoided eye contact with people staring at them through the glass wall. People standing outside creatively make up signs to perform visual conversations with friends and loved ones waiting in the inner part of the ward (over the reception desk).

In a constant game of negotiation, triage nurses try to maintain their authority to determine urgency. This authority is constantly interrupted and resisted by patients, as they attempt to gain attention and redirect its economy to their favor. Attention is a means of care that establishes worthiness and has an exchange value; it is also deployed among colleagues. Nurses do their best to justify their judgments, making them explicit in their written notes and actively making phone calls to doctors' internal offices to make them aware of the developing situations of patients waiting. In order to do their work, it is essential for nurses to manage people's long waits. This may trigger disputes or increase patients' suffering. In turn, doctors try to live up to the expectations of both patients and triage nurses, who often lobby to increase the speed of examinations during overcrowded shifts to alleviate suffering and avoid turmoil in the external waiting room.

This "struggle for visibility" involves the give and take of attention, and in the ER, it occurs in the midst of two different kinds of practical and temporal flow. On the one hand, patients wish to move from the periphery of the waiting room to the center of the ward where care is provided. To do so, they need to overcome material obstacles like the glass barrier and the fact that they have not yet been seen by triage nurses. Thus, they try to both get attention and position themselves in order to be noticed, forcing ER staff to acknowledge them and treat their distress.

On the other hand, health care providers want to focus on one task at a time. This involves withstanding the constant attempts by patients to move from the periphery to the center. From the nurses' point of view, incoming patients need to be managed and visitors positioned in space: they are either permitted to access internal offices or asked to wait patiently in the waiting room. Second, it means that nurses feel they need to control the ER's resources (medical examinations, ECGs and blood pressure cuffs, stretchers, wheelchairs, tests samples, work accident declarations, blood bags, dry ice, bandages, and so on). Third, nurses need to keep track of phone calls, including those from within the hospital (the inner side of the ER or other wards) asking about bureaucratic processes or demanding blood supplies or the direct fast-tracking of some patients.

Patients vie for nurses' attention during triage and doctors' attention later, during medical examinations. Attention is distributed by nurses by granting some patients some privacy and reevaluating others. Paying attention to complaining patients should ideally establish trust between the parties, ensuring a "compliant" relationship. But contrariwise, when a nurse feels mistreated by a patient's behavior, they tend to be more indifferent, which can give the patient the impression that the nurse is not paying attention and is not concerned with the patient's fate.

The experience of "not being seen," of not being the focus of a health care worker's attention, is dynamic and stratified. To those patients who already experience invisibility due to homelessness, xenophobia, or social abandonment, "not being seen" in the ER is both familiar and distressing.

The attention that nurses mobilize during their shifts depends on both inter-subjective processes and material conditions of health evaluations. Triage, as described, occurs in an open environment (glass wall and internal waiting room) where one cannot shut out distractions by simply closing a door, as in the office. Located between the waiting room and the doctor's office, triage is, in nurses' words, the "middle earth" (*la terra di mezzo*), "the port at sea" (*il porto di mare*) of the ER, where professionals feel stuck between patients' desires to get past the glass barrier and physicians' attempts to spend time evaluating patients and thus manage the waiting list according to their own schedule. Nurses describe their situation as being *tra l'incudine e il martello* (between the hammer and the anvil).

I started this chapter posing a question—Who decides when an urgent request for care is legitimate? How is such a decision made? The answer is that health care providers navigate triage assessment guidelines, contextualizing them in the rapidly changing environment of the ER, by weaving and managing particular economies of attention. Nurses shift between preestablished tasks to manage the habitual patterning of actions that support their work and by paying attention to newly emerging events that might always change their relations and their chances to craft urgency.

Urgency in the ER is not adjudicated; it is not based on fixed criteria of medical knowledge by a single expert decision-maker. Instead, urgency is a "routine of exceptions" (Lachenal, Lefève, and Nguyen 2014, 23–24), a constant compromise to navigate the tension between medical knowledge and social pressure, in which multiple actors influence triage outcomes. All this means that triage is anything but a clear-cut process of sorting. It emerges in the midst of a flow of resources, actors, and interactions and is negotiated in particular contexts. Attention circulates in the ER in ways that provide analytic traction to understand what happens there.

4 · CHANGING TIMES

Urgency in the ER is not only about bestowing and receiving attention—it is also about time. The assessment of patients' conditions by health care professionals and the attempts by patients and others to make themselves visible carve out particular configurations and experiences of time: they create temporalities. The plural is important here. More than one temporality coexists in the ER, and while often these different configurations and experiences of time harmonize, at other times, increasingly, they conflict.

A basic equation of time exists in the ER. To grant attention and urgency to something or someone, something else or someone else had to be made to wait. A complementary relation between urgency and waiting thus paced ER configuration and experiences of time. This balance was generally accepted, but it is always tenuous. It is threatened by a marketplace ethos in which patients are exhorted to see themselves as customers who should not have to wait to have their demand for services met but have no alternatives and no other place to go. The introduction of a marketplace ethos not only conflicted with the temporality of triage in the ER. It also fostered the influence of private interests over the state governance of public health care.

The temporality of urgency is a form of anticipation, which can be defined as "not just a reaction but a way of orienting oneself temporally" by organizing practice, material, and temporal arrangements in light of a forecasted future (Adams, Murphy, and Clarke 2009, 247). Determining urgency in the ER varied widely according to the ways that health care staff anticipated that people's cases would develop.

The internal offices of the ER—the ones on the internal side of the glass wall separating patients from medical staff—mirrored these variations. Each code had two dedicated offices. The offices for nonurgency white or low-priority green codes were relatively modest. There was a stretcher in the middle of the room, a long white desk and a sober black office chair, and a flat computer screen on the desk. An automated blood pressure cuff rested in the right corner beside a trolley full of single-use equipment like bandages, syringes, and plastic gloves.

The yellow-code area was equipped for high-risk priority cases. electrocardiogram (ECG) and ultrasound imaging machines were placed beside patients' stretchers, and intravenous painkillers were always within nurses' reach.

The red-code area was restricted to staff only, as opposed to the other three areas (yellow, green, and white) where each patient was allowed to be accompanied by one friend or relative, who could come into the office or wait just outside. In the red-code area, the wide range of medical equipment—sterile scalpels and gowns for surgery, instant casts, pumps, monitors detailing vital signs—was at medical staff's fingertips. There, bodies, often covered in blood, were incised and traversed by tubes and catheters. Bodies in trauma had precedence and dictated ER staff actions.

But while the ER was a place of urgency, it was also a place of often seemingly interminable waiting. Waiting constituted a different temporality and countered the idea of urgency. People waited multiple times in the ER: for a triage assessment, then for a doctor's examination, then for a specialist or a diagnostic test, then finally to be assigned a hospital bed or to receive a prescription for medications and be discharged from the ER. Health care professionals, too, waited in the ER: for patients and relatives to agree on a shared version of facts, for the results of diagnostic tests and specialists' consultations, and for the preannounced red codes to arrive in the ER by ambulance or helicopter transit.

In addition to the complementary relation between the fast-paced temporality of urgency and the more viscous temporality of waiting, a third temporality was increasingly present in the ER. This new way of regarding time was market-driven, embodied by patients and their friends and relatives who accompanied them, who increasingly took on the role of customers. This consumerist role was encouraged by the proclamations of private health care services and by shrill advertisements for medications that proclaimed to people that they did not deserve to wait nor should they be satisfied with a doctor's diagnosis if they felt they knew better. This new role for patients was one that eschewed waiting and demanded certainty. Challenging the ecology of time that oscillated between urgency and waiting in the ER and its inner rooms, consumer patients insisted on immediate certainty through concrete diagnostic tests such as ultrasound imaging, X-rays, and CAT (computerized axial tomography) scans.

Hence, in the ER governance over urgency was shaped by three coexisting temporalities: the assessment of risk by health care professionals, the experience of waiting by both those professionals and by patients, and the emerging challenge to this configuration by patients who, as paying customers, resisted waiting and wanted to decide for themselves how they should be examined and diagnosed. In contrast to the descriptions in the medical literature and in the professional education of triage, urgency in the ER was not a clear-cut decision-making process shaped by a biomedical framing of risks. It was much more complicated.

TIME IN THE ER: THE CASE OF SIGNOR STEFANO

8:06 p.m., a warm night of November—Thursday, night shift (8:00 p.m. to 7:00 a.m.)
I was shadowing Patrizia, a meticulous triage nurse in her late forties, in the internal waiting room at the ER. The place was crowded with people looking discouraged and bored, uncertain when their turn to see the doctor might arrive. The persistent ringing of the emergency phone punctuated the chatter of people waiting. Nurse Patrizia was reassuring an anxious woman in her sixties about her prolonged waiting when the ambulance arrived. Several volunteers and a nurse popped into the internal waiting area, escorting an overweight man in his mid-seventies who was sitting up straight on a stretcher, smiling. The ambulance crew stopped at the center of the internal waiting room, and Nurse Patrizia approached them.

The ambulance staff always presented triage nurses with a one-page form on which they reported their summary evaluation of possible risks. The form noted symptoms, pain severity, wounds, and the exact location of pain, indicated on a male silhouette used regardless of the patient's actual sex. The form also included personal data such as date of birth and address. This form was designed for acute cases such as car accidents or heart attacks, where the scene of the incident could be carefully recollected as could the moments before and immediately after the event, such as: Had the patient fainted? Is there any trauma to the skull? Does the patient respond to pain? What is the patient's state of consciousness?

This form from ambulance staff immediately set into motion a certain way of understanding time as "a photograph of the moment." This phrase *una fotografia del momento* was tirelessly repeated to training practitioners by triage nurses and ambulance staff. It indicated that a medical urgency contained everything that ER staff needed to know, in ways that could be objectified to fit the organizational structure of the ward.

In the case of the man who had just been brought in on the stretcher, however, nothing fit.

"We didn't get anything out of this one," a young nurse from the ambulance crew said, handing over to Nurse Patrizia the sheet with the man's vitals and personal data. "Signor Stefano was seen wandering around the city center without a destination. Some people passing by tried to question him and found he was confused and disoriented. So they called us. When we arrived, we found he spoke kind of slow, and he didn't seem to remember where he had parked his car."

The man, signor Stefano, sat on the stretcher staring at Nurse Patrizia, listening to the dialogue with a half-smile. He looked clumsy in his red-and-white flannel shirt, thick arms, and tousled silver hair.

"He has not fainted and seems just to be a little bradycardic [he has a slow heartbeat rate], but who knows!" the ambulance nurse continued, using the Italian expression *Boh!*, meaning "It's anyone's guess." "Initially, he didn't want to come along to the hospital. We had to convince him to get a checkup. That's all.

Hope you get more out of him!" The ambulance crew turned and left, leaving Nurse Patrizia to turn to her new patient.

"Signor Stefano, what happened?" she said in a friendly tone.

"I don't know. . . . You tell me," he replied slowly, in a deep baritone.

"Do you feel a little confused? What do you remember?"

"I was going to visit my sister who lives in the city center, but she wasn't home. So I walked back to the car but, for a moment, I didn't remember where it was. So a couple of guys helped me out."

"How did you feel back then? And how are you now?"

"I'm fine. They said I was confused, but I am just fine."

Nurse Patrizia winced, not at all convinced that he was "just fine," and she walked away to get the blood pressure monitor and the ECG machine. After taking some vitals, she evaluated for possible neurological damage by testing her new patient's state of consciousness and orientation in time and space.

"Signor Stefano, where are we?" she began.

"In the hospital. Right?" he replied, annoyed.

"Yes. In which year?"

"Mmmh, 2017," he said, staring at Nurse Patrizia like she was an extraterrestrial alien.

"Good. Month?"

"Mmmh . . . September!" Actually, it was already the first week of November, but the weather was warm and sunny, not unlike a typical September day.

"Mmmh," Nurse Patrizia nodded, wincing again. She seemed to have found what she was looking for.

"Do you remember where you parked?" she asked.

"Actually, now I do," signor Stefano replied. "Can I go now?"

Signor Stefano seemed not to realize that he had been taken by ambulance fifteen kilometers from the city center. It was the middle of the night, so no buses were running. It later transpired that he had no money for a cab.

"No," said Nurse Patrizia, with a reassuring smile. "Now we need to see what happened. We need to be sure that everything is fine. Let me put your data into our computer. The doctor will soon call you for your examination. By the way, can I have your sister's phone number?"

Nurse Patrizia and I left signor Stefano in a cubicle in the inner waiting area. The anxious woman whom she had been speaking to when signor Stefano was brought in was screaming loudly: "I've waited long enough!" Nurse Patrizia ignored her.

Behind the glass barrier of the reception desk, she looked up signor Stefano's medical records. They revealed that he had suffered from a major period of depression and was still receiving treatment at a local mental health service.

The ER database that Nurse Patrizia had checked was organized in a way that allowed practitioners to connect people's legal identity and frame their situation in time through their triage assessment form (present situation) and their medical records (past medical history) to more accurately estimate the urgency of their treatment (i.e., the future). The database was an internal network accessible only to hospital staff. Data were collected from the ER over time and shared among linked wards in the same hospital, including, for example, psychiatry, neurology, the intensive care unit, and urology. The network data, however, usually did not include GPs' prescriptions, external specialists' examinations, or medical charts from other hospitals. The absence of all relevant information complicated the assessment of a given patient.

Documents play an important role in shaping time and objects of knowledge in the clinic, as medical anthropologists and sociologists have described.[1] In the ER computer program, waiting and urgency constantly constitute each other. Nurse Patrizia, after having her perception mediated by the "ambulance patients' form," needed to type into the computer system her evaluation by anticipating biological risks so that the software could rearrange the list of people waiting after the new open case, signaling a new ranking of urgency to doctors in the internal ER offices.

"He might have been having a psychotic crisis," Nurse Patrizia conjectured about her new patient. "But, more likely, it was a transient global state of confusion or a TIA [transient ischemic attack, a minor stroke], which is not a good sign," she explained to me as she filled out the triage form, typing it out on the computer. "He looks bad [è brutto]. Better go for a yellow code."

As I noted in chapter 3, in ER jargon looking "bad" means that medical staff suspect that "something" might be going on inside a patient's body. Saying that someone "looks bad" means both that the health care provider is uncertain about the patient's situation and also that they have a "bad" feeling about it. Such a feeling already configured a progressive motion, a developing pathological time.

After taking several emergency calls about incoming patients with red codes, Nurse Patrizia rang signor Stefano's sister, who was the person listed on his ambulance form as his next of kin. The woman answered at the third attempt.

"No, I am not coming to collect him!" she said when Nurse Patrizia explained the purpose of her call. "I have to get up early for work tomorrow! We live in the mountains and it takes an hour to drive there and another to get back! He is always playing these tricks on us! We cannot let our lives be destroyed because he is f-cking depressed!"

With the end of the call, clear that signor Stefano was on his own, Nurse Patrizia tried to fast-track his case into the doctor's office.

I escorted signor Stefano into the doctor's office while Nurse Patrizia remained in the triage area. The doctor on duty that night, a woman in her thirties named Elena, started by asking signor Stefano the same questions Patrizia had asked. Signor Stefano gave almost the same answers. This is not always the case. At times, health care providers complain that people change their versions of facts according to whom they speak. Memory and perception are not crystallized in people's minds, and changes occur according to context and the habit of expressing what issue is at stake. A lamented tendency is that people exaggerate their stress and pain in the triage area in order to get access to the doctor's office. Once they are with the doctor, patients tend to elaborate more on their condition and are generally more compliant, mindful that the power imbalance between participants has increased but also because the doctor's office is a closed space. A trusting relationship can be more easily established.

When it came to naming the month, signor Stefano said, "Mmmh . . . October? Everyone keeps asking me, so I must have got it wrong."

After a few more questions, the doctor said, "Well, let's call your sister again, shall we?" His sister answered and repeated her refusal to come and pick up her brother from the hospital. "Can he just stay for the night?" she asked. "Tomorrow I will come by to get him. Can you just admit him into any ward?"

"Signora, this is a hospital, not a hotel!" said Dr. Elena, flinging down the receiver. The doctor prescribed CAT to confirm Nurse Patrizia's diagnosis that signor Stefano may have suffered a minor stroke and to check if it had left any brain damage. An hour later, the CAT turned out negative.

When signor Stefano returned to her office, Dr. Elena said to him: "Let's talk to someone, huh?"

He nodded. Dr. Elena rang the psychiatric ward. A few minutes later, a young psychiatrist, Dr. Natalia, arrived. Dr. Natalia addressed signor Stefano in a gentle tone, inviting him to follow her to another office in the yellow-code area and then to sit on the stretcher as he pleased. He clearly welcomed the invitation to sit comfortably, and he began to speak freely about his situation. I stood next to Dr. Natalia during the interview while Dr. Elena moved on to examine other patients. We discovered that signor Stefano lived alone in a small village in the Apennines. His sister—the one the hospital staff had been calling—lived in the mountains near signor Stefano, but they had a difficult relationship. He felt very lonely at times, and whenever this happened, he would drive into the city to meet his other deaf sister, who lived in the city center.

Upon concluding this brief interview, the psychiatrist turned to Dr. Elena and told her that she could not find anything wrong with signor Stefano. Hearing this, signor Stefano perked up. "So can I go now?" he asked. "It's already 4:00 A.M. Can I go get my car?"

At this point, it was ascertained that signor Stefano had no money to pay for a taxi back into town. "The best we can do," Dr. Elena said, "is to try and call your sister again." She called again and the sister argued with her. Finally, faced with the threat of the hospital suing her for abandoning a vulnerable elderly person, the sister finally agreed to come and get signor Stefano.

She arrived an hour and a half later, at 6:30 A.M. She strode up to signor Stefano and, with a disgusted expression, barked, "You always mess everything up. Now just get up and let's go!"

RATING RISK: TIME IN THE EXAMINATION AREA

The different approaches to signor Stefano's situation and the forms of subjectivity—in the sense of personhood and organization of experience that resulted from those different approaches—illuminate how time in the ER is created by pacing the risk-rating process (Biehl, Good, and Kleinman 2007). The making of clinical urgency aims to identify and thus enact in practice risks embedded in bodily conditions (Mol 2002). What this means in practice is that people, technology, and bodies need to be organized in the ER so that their relation allows health care providers to successfully craft urgency and so pace the ward activities. This process is understood by ER staff as not aiming at diagnostic certainty but as a good enough pathway to tackle immediate bodily developments.

Risk rating in the ER differs from what usually happens in other wards of the hospital. As Annemarie Mol describes in her work on atherosclerosis (a disease of the arteries) in a Dutch hospital, time is structured around different ways of engaging and revealing disease through the different approaches it receives in surgery, radiology, and internal medicine wards (2002, 4–12). Disease as a unique and "multiple" object at once directs surgeons' incisions in the operating theater. Similarly, enactments of disease affect the time of diagnostic imaging. They pace medical ward activities through, say, recordkeeping and drug intake (68–70).

In contrast, the anthropologist Alice Street describes how doctors' actions in the hospital in Madang, Papua New Guinea, were "not dependent on specific enactments of disease" (2011b, 824; 2014). "Instead, action was correlated with what was feasible" (824). Detailing the harsh shortages of this hospital, Street shows that at the center of health professionals' concerns is which treatment options are available, not the "revelation of disease" through technologies of visibility, such as X-ray imaging or ultrasounds (825). To face resource shortages in Madang, efforts were focused on fashioning "relationships between persons, technologies and bodies in order to direct a patient's trajectory away from death and towards discharge" (831). Time was not structured around disease, as in Mol's case. Instead, temporality progressed through the "opening and closing" of practical pathways of intervention, those that determined forms of personhood such as the division between "generically sick patients" and those who received treatment by doctors (825).

Even though the situation of the hospital where I did my fieldwork is significantly different from the one Street describes in Madang, the triage of medical attention that she highlights resembles the way time was structured in the ER. The opening and closing of practical pathways relates to how nurses and doctors in the ER often explained triage and risk rating (i.e., urgency) by contrasting them with a diagnosis. Diagnosis was a medical label that was already shaped and imagined as a more or less stable temporal entity. "Someone might have cancer but not be coded as an urgency in the ER," nurses explained to waiting patients, because cancer is not usually immediately life threatening. Urgency, on the other hand, was a rapidly emerging process to be assessed and treated.

The fluidity and instability of clinical urgency is evident in the pacing of signor Stefano's case. When he arrived in the ER in an ambulance, he was classified as a vulnerable, deserving subject with a "high priority," even though he claimed to feel fine and just wanted to go home. It subsequently took six hours to exclude possible biomedical risk factors. During this time, health professionals tried to detect whether anything was acting beneath his body's surface that they could prioritize as a "real," urgent threat.

By doing so, they did not aim primarily at objectifying signor Stefano's situation through a specific diagnostic label (for instance, as a cancer patient or a heart attack victim) but at producing a form of personhood and organized experience of subjectivity to enable the staff to anticipate risk. Color codes like the yellow code that signor Stefano was given by Nurse Patrizia immediately made different degrees of risk visible, and health care providers used them to readily distinguish between patients who needed immediate attention and those who could wait.

The ER staff's constant concern to anticipate risks and urgent developments in patients' conditions paced time in the ER. As the anthropologist Cheryl Mattingly noticed within clinical practice, actions are organized to carve out "plots" to build familiar narratives that enable a sense of time and therapeutic progression and ultimately hope and healing (1994, 811–812; 1998; 2009). Time is not linear but is dependent on negotiation in a context amid the diverse motives of actors, in which improvisation plays a significant role in its structuring and experience (Mattingly 1994, 820).

Within the ER, too, time can be analyzed as punctuated by shifting therapeutic horizons. But rather than thinking of ER time as a structure of linear progression, it seems more fruitful to think of it in terms of an ecosystem, one that ebbs and flows between the rapid pacing of urgency and a slow, sometimes seemingly infinite time of waiting.

For signor Stefano, three main moments scaled up urgency and turned time toward waiting: (1) the initial urgent search for medical risks, (2) the psychiatric evaluation slowing down the interaction, and (3) the retreat of a biomedical focus on signor Stefano's bodily condition and the acknowledgment of other grounds of action that were related to his life. These grounds resulted in health care providers waiting for signor Stefano's sister to arrive at the ER to pick him up.

The ER staff focus was initially directed toward signor Stefano's apparent confusion and slowness and a possible minor stroke. The staff read bodily signs as effects of internal actors (blood, vessels, the heart's electrical activity, cognitive functioning). An escalating temporality of urgency emerged as signor Stefano's looking "bad," resulting in his swift admission into the ER. It lost its traction when the diagnostic attempts to pinpoint medical causes were unsuccessful.

When that happened, Dr. Elena decided to order a psychiatric evaluation. This slowed down time. Once it was established that signor Stefano had not had a minor stroke, the segmentation of time expanded, turning from a rapidly paced urgency to a more moderately paced rhythm, during which the psychiatric intervention could unfold. Dr. Natalia, the psychiatrist, approached signor Stefano with a set of questions that opened up space for other ways of understanding his situation. "Do you live alone? What do you do in your spare time? Who comes to visit you? How often?" These questions allowed the relations that made up signor Stefano's life, his loneliness and feelings of abandonment, to come into focus as relevant for handling his situation in the ER. This again changed the way time was paced, turning further away from urgency and shaping a temporality that ultimately resulted in Dr. Elena waiting for signor Stefano's sister to come to the ER and collect him. By calling signor Stefano's sister multiple times, including to emphasize that the hospital was not a hotel, Dr. Elena reaffirmed her authority to determine the definition of what was urgent and what could wait.

Urgency and waiting are not opposites in the ER. They are not two sides of one coin. Instead, they complement each other. Waiting coexisted constantly with urgency in health care providers' routines. Dr. Elena had to wait for signor Stefano to make sense so that she could decide what to do. Then she had to wait for the result of signor Stefano's CAT scan and for the psychiatrist to come downstairs to the ER to make her evaluation. Waiting allowed practitioners to gather data and prioritize tasks, thereby enabling them to make decisions about urgency. Urgency could unfold only because something else could be made to wait.

The kind of attention that signor Stefano was given in the ER is a limited resource. Health professionals perceive urgency as having a quick tempo, as an acute and measurable crisis that requires immediate intervention. Other dimensions of people's lives that do not constitute a helpful pathway to address clinical urgency are usually bracketed out of interactions. Those other dimensions of people's lives are directed to a specific place and a specific temporality—namely, the waiting room where they wait.

WAITING IN THE ER

Anyone who comes to the ER on their own—that is, who is not brought there in an ambulance or a helicopter—likely spends most of their time in the waiting room. In the hospital where I worked, this is a square space with no window, with seats molded together in rows. The number of seats is usually sufficient for patients, but many individuals are too anxious to sit. They stand or walk back and forth between the row of seats and the glass wall that separates the waiting room from the examination rooms.

While in the red-code area, people's bodies turn into a battleground of professionals' efforts—naked, separated from relatives and friends, cut open, traversed by tubes and catheters. From the waiting room, one cannot see what happens inside the inner sections of the ER where ambulances arrive. Only the helicopter's roar can be heard approaching the red-code area, where the absolute now of biology is unleashed and painkillers, blood thinners, antibodies, and blood bags swirl like a cocktail mix within veins. In the waiting room, people are just left wondering what happens inside.

People who came to the ER arrived knowing that they were likely to wait. They came equipped with newspapers (the few that the hospital staff deposit in the waiting room—*la Repubblica* and *la Gazzetta dello Sport*—are usually too well-thumbed to be particularly appealing), magazines, novels, smartphones, and laptops, although power outlets were few and the object of frequent conflicts. Families with children brought toys and video games. Some stared at the flat TV screen, turned to a quiet volume and set in the upper-left corner of the room, which mostly showed news and weather broadcasts and local nursing home and heath care–related commercials. Many people settled in for the wait with water bottles and snacks brought from home or purchased at vending machines in the ER waiting room. More experienced visitors to the ER sometimes came bearing a bag with pajamas, anticipating that they might be admitted for the night.

Waiting here was a slow affair. The only thing that gave a sense of time passing was nurses summoning patients through the raspy loudspeaker behind the glass wall. Attention to these calls was crucial: names were only repeated twice, and if you missed your call, you lost your spot on the waiting list.

When I asked people in the waiting room to talk about their experience of waiting, many told me *è un grande mistero* (it's a great mystery). They felt they had no control over how long they had to wait and what to expect next. The absence of reference points and information was disorienting. Although I was not a waiting patient, I could not help notice how different time felt in the waiting room compared to the rapid pace of action and care that occurred on the other side of the glass barrier. The paradox of sitting in the waiting room, as often pointed out to me by patients, was to feel simultaneously unattended, invisible, yet also constantly surveilled. The institutional space and the wide glass wall that divided it from the rest of the ward was experienced as a kind of panoptic structure, and it instilled in waiting patients (and in staff: recall the aquarium metaphor) a sense of being scrutinized (Foucault 1991a).

In this situation, waiting can be illuminated by the work of the sociologist Javier Auyero (2012), who writes of waiting rooms in welfare and state administrative offices in Buenos Aires, Argentina. Drawing on Foucault's understanding of power as both repressive and productive, Auyero discusses waiting as a disciplinary practice that transforms people into docile state subjects—"patients of the state," whose time is disposable in relation to state bureaucratic procedures (2012, 3, 7–14; Foucault 1991a).

Auyero's "patient" metaphor, of course, is not just metaphor in the ER. In the ER, the disciplinary dimension of waiting was underscored by making it "a great mystery" through the absence of information and time references. However, the productive side of normalizing waiting and of making people into subjects whose time was determined by forces and decisions beyond their knowledge or control was not accepted by everyone. The time spent waiting was not simply passively suffered; it was oftentimes also "actively" used.

The anthropologist Clara Han describes how women from heavily indebted families in Santiago, Chile, found ways to exert agency through what she calls "active waiting": allowing time to pass as a means of care for themselves and others (Han 2011, 26; 2012; cf. Brown 2012). Han describes waiting as a site of emerging possibilities that needed to be strategically crafted and upheld (2011, 25). Similarly, in the ER people carved out time from other necessities and obligations to stand the long waits, coordinating efforts through texts and phone calls with families and friends to, say, fetch basic goods like foods and water, exchange advice, and keep each other company. In the ER where I worked, some patients, through what Han calls active waiting, did not become docile state subjects. They strategically used their waiting to reshape their time.

An example was signor Ahmad—a skinny thirty-two-year-old man with curly Afroed hair poking out from his worn-out red baseball cap. He had recently been evicted from his apartment, and he was waiting for the second time in three days in the ER. Soon after we spoke, he had to leave the ER, giving up his spot on the waiting list to avoid missing the appointment he had with a social worker who was helping him find shelter for the night. After arranging this meeting, which he did by texting the social services office repeatedly from the ER waiting room, signor Ahmad decided that he could afford to ignore his sudden partial facial paralysis (caused either by sleeping out in the cold or by a damaged nerve or, perhaps, by both) because he felt that his more urgent need was to find shelter to sleep properly, shower, and try his luck with job interviews. He left me. saying "It doesn't matter. I will come back to the ER a third time."

Another example was signora Rita, an animated woman of about fifty, dressed in a vivid scarlet jacket. Due to a fall a month earlier, she had a swollen foot with a wide purple cut that meant she could barely walk. Signora Rita told me that she had wanted to come to the ER ever since her fall but she was not able to because her fifteen-year-old son had a disability, and he could not be left alone. She was his only support. After lengthy negotiations, she was able to get her neighbor to look after him while she went to the ER. She had left home at 5:00 A.M., hoping to make it back in time for her neighbor to go to work. As it turned out, though, it was already midday, and she was still waiting. She spent her time anxiously texting on WhatsApp to check on the situation at home and intermittently looking up, hoping to hear her name called.

Active waiting highlights the trade-off that is the implicit bargain offered by the ER. The time that patients waited was equally distributed according to practices of biomedical risk rating. All green-coded patients, for example, were expected to endure more or less the same amount of waiting. But as the examples of signor Ahmed and signora Rita indicate, waiting was related not just to biomedical risk rating. Whether people waited, and how, was linked to concerns and obligations far outside the ER—the need to care for a loved one, the necessity of finding a place to spend the night, dealing with other state apparatuses (like welfare services or the police), and the obligation to go back to work. What the above examples show is how people actively rearranged their time in order to wait in the ER for the possibility of medical attention.

In the examples of signor Ahmed and signora Rita, the experience of waiting time was more active than it was passive, but they also illustrate that the essential configuration of time in the ER was left untouched. Through active waiting, patients occupied their time in what for them were relatively productive ways. But those activities did not change the authority that health care providers had to define what and who should wait and what and who should be attended to first. On the contrary. Through practices of active waiting, the time balance between urgency and waiting was upheld.

Unsettling the time balance between urgency and waiting, however, was a relatively new temporality, linked to and driven by the market-driven sense of entitlement that some patients assumed. For those individuals, time in the ER, rather than oscillating between urgency and waiting, was imagined to be propelled by demands that should swiftly be followed by gratification. This orientation toward time involved a disdain for waiting and a reframing of individuals from being patients who were compelled to wait to being fee-for-service customers whose demands should be quickly satisfied.

THE TIME OF FEE-FOR-SERVICE

A good emergency worker does not provide a diagnosis.

Like a mantra, this phrase was tirelessly repeated when nurses explained to me and others what it is that they and emergency doctors did in the ER. Risk assessment was not about certainty, this mantra affirmed; it was about perceiving possibilities. Urgency was about sorting options, not revealing the definitive shape of disease. A more precise approximation of people's conditions could only be reached at a later stage, once diagnostic tests had been performed, after urgency.

Doctors tried to pin down a specific diagnosis in the ER and sometimes ordered extensive technological examinations (ECGs, blood tests, X-rays, CAT scans, or MRIs) due to the insistent request of an anxious patient or out of personal curiosity or professional concern at missing "something." Those who did so were not well thought of among nurses. Such inquisitive physicians were half-jokingly called "the scientists" (*gli scienziati*). The term was pejorative: it implied that the doctor in question could not deal with uncertainty. The older generation of nurses, like Nurse Patrizia, were particularly quick to label doctors in this way. Patrizia was in her forties, and she did not have university-based training (which was only introduced in Italy in 1995; see Saiani 2016). She and other nurses of her generation and older had learned from experience how to properly "sense danger" at first sight. These nurses walked a thin line between official guidelines and experiential authority.

This generation of nurses in particular—giving voice to a widespread sentiment among all ER staff—felt that patients who increasingly asked for diagnostic tests were a threat to their profession. Phrases like "I pay your salary with my taxes, so I am your boss" (Pago il tuo stipendio con le tasse quindi sono il tuo capo) were widely shared among nurses and the most experienced physicians to mimic the sense of entitlement that they felt rising among patients.

The neoliberal reform of 1992, which reorganized public hospitals and regional and local health units into private enterprises, made hospitals accountable for meeting budget targets and responsible for customer satisfaction. Prior to 1994, a reimbursement system based on hospital yearly expenditures—cost-based payment—was at play. However, in 1994, Italy's National Health Service introduced a new financial system to reduce expenditures. The system was based on payments for fixed costs related to particular diagnostic procedures (Diagnostic-Related Group [DRG], calculated according to the International Classification of Diseases, ICD-9), such as surgery, pharmaceuticals, diagnostic examinations, and professionals' work (Comodo and Maciocco 2011, 70–71).

This meant that the more diagnoses a hospital made, the more money a hospital administration would receive from regional authorities financed by the state. The DRG system calculates diagnosis costs for each ward over each patient discharged after a hospital stay. ERs, however, are not financed through the DRG system (Ameri, Cremonesi, and Montefiori 2011). Hospital administrations instead reimburse ERs on the basis of the previous year's expenditures (i.e., retaining a cost-based payment).

The important difference here is that an ER's financial budget is fixed. It does not increase annually, as it is not based on an ER's increasing care activity. It thus cannot possibly cover the skyrocketing costs of ER overcrowding and the increasing requests for care from an always more precarious population. The ER became in effect a financial sinkhole once the DRG system was implemented, while wards like internal medicine, cardiology, and others became diagnosis "production machines," highly profitable for a hospital structure (Meng et al. 2020).

These same conditions also applied to private practice, which was developing, even flourishing, as a relatively new market. Private and public health care were given similar footing by the state, and diagnoses became products to be sold. Leaving financial sinkholes like the ER to the public system, private practices could focus on profitable health care services like specialist outpatient clinics, diagnostic exams, or residential older adult care homes. The DRG system created a strong competitive advantage for private structures that were now being paid by both the Italian state and by patients for their services.

As a result of this reform in 1994, private insurance and pharmaceutical companies began heavily investing in advertising that portrayed care as driven by demand. They promoted an understanding of medical services as customer centered, with concern focused on patients' choices rather than needs (Mol 2008). Addressing the problem of patient choice in a Dutch diabetes outpatient service, Annemarie Mol (2008, 25) suggests that in order to feed the market, seductive marketing strategies fuel individual desire for health care. They encourage independent patient choices, but ultimately, they only foster an "illusion of control," replacing professional counseling and careful reasoning with a lonely customer-centered kind of decision-making based on superficial desire (25–26).

In the ER, this ethos collided with what emergency workers envisioned as their duty. An immediate effect of this was the increasingly frequent conflicts between reluctant health care providers and people taking on the role of customer. Staff in the ER agreed that the most difficult patients were the ones who behaved like customers and who treated the ER staff as though they were shop assistants.

A young ER physician named Paolo illustrated this to me in a story about an incident that had occurred a few days previously.

It was a Saturday morning, and things were going quite well at work. We had an adequate workforce for once: we were very near to the famous zero-list [no patients on the waiting list]. I let the next patient in. The triage note said, "Just seen by the doctor on call [*guardia medica*], in a place nearby. Pain at hips and when urinating. Kidney stone? Cystitis? Woman age 24, no critical situation." She was registered in the system and walked into my office eight or nine minutes later. Her name was Maria, and she was accompanied by her mother, signora Gianna, because, as you know, here it's the norm to let relatives into the office.[2] It was one of those days I felt kind of nice [*ero di buona*]. I asked Maria what was wrong, and she replied that it burned when she peed. I asked again if it had happened before, and she said no, and no allergies to medications either. . . . In short: straightforward case.

At that point, I thought that the local doctor on call had not quite done her job [*nullafacente*], so I asked her to see the medical report the doctor had given her. I can assure you that I've never seen a better written report. A young colleague doing a beautiful cystitis report complete with meds prescriptions. It was dated sixty minutes earlier in a place forty minutes away from the ER. So, I stood there, surprised and confused. The doctor on call had rightly prescribed analgesic therapy and an antibiotic and also some sort of follow-up visit, which by the way never happens! She gave specific instructions of what to do.

So I asked Maria what had happened during the time that had elapsed. "Did you get an allergic reaction from the antibiotic?" Her mother, signora Gianna, answered. "No, no," she told me. "We came here straight from the clinic."

"But, why? Is she getting worse? A slight temperature is normal . . ."

I noticed that signora Gianna was addressing me with a "we" to speak for her daughter, even though her daughter was an adult woman of twenty-four, perfectly sane and lucid. She told me that "they" had not taken the antibiotic because "they" did not trust the doctor on call.

"Why don't you trust her" I asked, and I explained that she was a very efficient colleague. She had done her job beautifully. But the mother was not convinced.

"She was too young," signora Gianna said. I checked the doctor's *codice fiscale* [social security number], and she was born in '89. I was born in '88.

"Look," I said, "I am only eleven months older than her." The tone between us was still friendly.

"I thought the problem was merely a prejudice the signora had." Dr. Paolo told me he confirmed the other doctor's diagnosis and encouraged Maria to take the prescribed antibiotic as soon as possible.

This upset her mother, who barked, "What?! You're not even going to give her an ultrasound?"

As nicely as I could, I said, "It can be helpful, but now there is nothing indicating that we should do it. The doctor on call recommended it in her report if the symptoms don't go away. But we are talking about two or three days from now, after we see if the medication works."

"At least take a urine culture!" the mother insisted.[3]

"That isn't necessary either, signora," I said. "Only in case she doesn't improve."

"So you're not doing anything!"

"It's not that I'm not doing anything; it's just that everything has already been done," I replied. "Look signora, let's close it down here." But I also dared to try to lecture her, thinking of the next time she would want to take her daughter to the ER: "I don't think it's right to come to the ER for such a small thing, and you have to know that." Signora Gianna jumped up from the chair, but I continued:

"It's wrong for three reasons. Today it went well, but she could have been forced to wait six hours, to use the restroom in the waiting area, and to pay the fee for misuse of the ER."

She shouted, "You think I care?! It's only twenty-five euros!"

"But it is also a cost for the community," I replied, as courteously as I could.

But then she got arrogant. "Sure! It will be because of my misuse that the health system goes bankrupt!"

At that point, I started treating her like a moron by telling her that the principle is the same as: I do not throw trash on the ground because, if we all did, the world would be inundated by trash. On top of all this, while I spoke, signora Gianna called me *tu* without any deference, while I was still using *lei* to address her.[4]

And then she got agitated: "Cut the bullshit—we've already understood that you don't wanna do shit!"

I was outraged and I ordered her to get out of the office so that I could finish the examination just with her daughter, who, unfortunately, was not that different from her mother. I told the daughter that I was sorry if she was discontent with the outcome of the examination, but I couldn't do more than that. I thought it would end there. Just an everyday encounter with an idiot. To me, people like them are part of those antivax movements and Grillini [the populist antiestablishment Italian party Five Star Movement]. I've gotten used to them.

NO WAITING

What provoked Dr. Paolo most about his encounter with signora Gianna and her daughter Maria was not the mother's arrogance and disrespect but the way she treated the ER as a kind of shopping experience whose raison d'être was to service her desires. She acted like a customer, insisting on more tests to determine her daughter's problem even though a path of care had already been determined (expertly, in Dr. Paolo's view). Signora Gianna declared that she had not trusted the doctor on call, and she made it equally clear that she regarded Dr. Paolo as incompetent and obstructionist.

What seemed to be at stake for signora Gianna was her capacity to determine her daughter's care in order to provide immediate medical recognition of her daughter's suffering—which an ultrasound might bestow—and perhaps also to enact her role as a "caring mother" (Whyte, van der Geest, and Hardon 2003, 23–36). Her capacity to "do something" about her daughter's suffering, by this logic, was blocked by Dr. Paolo when he denied her a more extensive diagnostic examination. The unfolding of time in care delivery was to signora Gianna clearly to be driven by her demands, as a paying customer. For her, this implied that she should not be made to wait.

Dr. Paolo was of another view. He interpreted signora Gianna's behavior as an irresponsible expression of selfishness in relation to the public collective and a waste of tax-payers' money. He remarked later in our conversation that

> usually, these kinds of patients aren't low class, but middle or upper class. They are arrogant toward institutions, challenging and threatening. You can recognize them by the way they go into the ER, treating the staff as if they were mechanics at a car repair workshop. They presume they know everything and are hyperaggressive. They want diagnostic examinations but don't follow medical advice. They don't want to wait; they just want the tests. I'll quote my mentor: an X-ray never cured anyone.

While even if an X-ray never cured anyone, examinations involving concrete tests like X-rays, or the ultrasound demanded by signora Gianna, were marketed continuously by television, newspapers, and online commercials as the instant solution to people's uncertain health conditions. Immediate certainty and a rapid service delivery were at the center of private insurance and pharmaceutical companies' campaigns that recommended abundant screenings, specialist consultations, and other medical tests that had been turned into sellable commodities.

Such tendencies reflect a more general trend in Italy. As the anthropologist Andrea Muehlebach (2012) describes, after the financial collapse of 2008 people in Italy fell prey to a powerful existential crisis. In response, certainty was turned into a key mediatic device to counter anxieties toward an uncertain future. Biomedical sensemaking, in particular, became a language that in the eyes of many could provide a much-desired certainty of outcome.

Contrary to the long waiting lists of the public services, private campaigns and commercials all but erased waiting from the picture. The emphasis, instead, was on immediate satisfaction and unequivocal certainty—something that allegedly resulted from technical diagnostic tests (Mol 2008, 18–23). Rather than an ecosystem of time that ebbed and flowed between urgency and waiting, market-driven temporality connected demand directly with gratification. There was no space—and no time—for waiting.

As this temporality of consumption becomes increasingly entrenched in people's understanding of what medical services are for, it is perhaps unsurprising that people like signora Gianna feel entitled to determine care on the basis of demand. Drawing from a market-driven fantasy of immediate therapeutic intervention, signora Gianna was not willing to "wait and see" as Dr. Paolo proposed.[5] She wanted an instant unequivocal outcome, and she wanted it on demand. "Not doing shit" was an affront to her.

Dr. Paolo's encounter with signora Gianna did not end when her daughter Maria left his office. When he stepped out into the triage area, he saw that signora

Gianna was "raising hell" (*fare il diavolo a quattro*) with nurses, in front of all the waiting patients. As soon as signora Gianna saw Dr. Paolo, she threatened him, shouting that she knew his name and that she would sue. Dr. Paolo felt that with that threat, signora Gianna had crossed a line, and he decided to fight back. He ordered signora Gianna to give him a valid identification document. She refused, even though to refuse was to commit a criminal offense since Dr. Paolo was a public officer on duty.[6] He called the hospital guards and then reported her to the police in order to sue her for interruption of public service, offense, and threatening (*oltraggio e minaccia*) a public officer.

After the *denucia* (police report) was filed with the police officer on call, one of Dr. Paolo's colleagues, a senior physician, came out of his inner office and tried to calm signora Gianna down by registering her daughter in the ER system once again. "As if nothing had happened," Dr. Paolo told me.

"And he let her have every useless test she demanded," he continued. "He [the senior physician] did this in good faith [*in buona fede*], and he was doing it to protect me, but I felt belittled nevertheless. I wanted him to take a stand [as a professional]."

The senior doctor also told signora Gianna that she did not have to pay the fine for misusing the ER that Dr. Paolo had issued, "in order to avoid further fuss."

Dr. Paolo told me that he was supported by the nurses and the *operatore socio-sanitario* (OSS) personnel (sociomedical aid workers), but only a few other physicians expressed their solidarity. His conclusion was that because the ongoing processes of neoliberalization of the health care service made their jobs increasingly precarious, health professionals did not feel safe confronting patients who assumed the unsatisfied customer role. Instead, many simply acquiesced in response to being bullied by patients like signora Gianna. Although other physicians agreed with Dr. Paolo that a fee-for-service temporality based on customer demands cannot determine how the ER is run, "they just didn't have the guts to express their dissent with the current state of things."

"Also," he said, "the hospital administration [Direzione Sanitaria] kept quiet. I wasn't expecting a medal, but at least something! 'These are things that we see every day,' I told them. 'Aren't you tired of it?' And I received a deafening silence in return. I got scared and looked for answers, reaching out to some of the hospital's executive managers, trying to figure out what was next for me. I felt very much alone even though I thought that I had both law and reason on my side. My case went out on all news and social networks. After a while, I got some support from the hospital administration board. But I wanted to convey a different message, something more than could be communicated by merely issuing a fine to that signora.

"Staremo a vedere" (We will see), he concluded his story to me gravely.

As far as I know, the lawsuit against signora Gianna never made it to court. But I do know that Dr. Paolo's contract at the ER was not renewed.

CHANGING TIMES IN THE ER

In exploring the role of time in defining urgency in the ER, we have seen how the temporalities of clinical urgency, waiting, and fee-for-service consumerism coexist. But they differ in an important way. Urgency and waiting, together, constitute different dimensions of the same temporal ecosystem. Together they structure and pace the activities that take place in the ER. A crucial part of the negotiation of urgency involves the boundary between the examination room and the waiting room. This distinction is both based on and enabled by the asymmetry of power and expertise between patients and ER staff. It permits health care providers to prioritize relations and actions or delay them in time.

The temporal dimension of waiting, unsurprisingly, was felt most acutely in the waiting room. There, patients felt absorbed by a "great mystery," not knowing when their name would be called. Many patients accepted the need to wait, as already described. They found ways to make that time "active," using it to care for others, texting and calling friends or social workers, and occupying themselves with snacks, conversations, magazines, and smartphones. These activities made the experience of waiting more bearable and enjoyable, but importantly, they facilitated the maintenance of the strict division between the waiting room and the examination area, between waiting and urgency.

What unsettled the key role of waiting, threatening to radically transform the way in which care and time are governed in the ER, was the market-driven temporality of fee-for-service consumers. This newly emerging way of thinking about health care compelled patients to think of the ER as a service that they could demand, on their own terms. This attitude threatened the health care providers' ability to manage the economy of attention that sustained their work.

Creating the subjectivity of the unsatisfied customer, private practices and insurance introduced another way to govern care in the ER that is not based on triage as a form of gatekeeping. The subjectivity of the customer changes the distribution of care required by patients. As Gianna and Maria's case illustrates, new requests for care often resulted in conflicts that drastically changed how care is administered by the ER and governmentality is enacted by the Italian state.

Yet the increasing requests to the ER for help are not only tied to the relentless advertisements of the private health sector. As I will show in chapter 5, it is instead the direct support the Italian state provides to market interests that creates the controversial category of the so-called inappropriate users.

5 · TRIAGE AT AN IMPASSE
Making "Inappropriate Users"

> To expect short waiting times from the underfunded ER without increasing resources is like sticking a Ferrari logo on a Panda [economy car produced by FIAT] and hoping it will run 280km/h!
> —Facebook post by a triage nurse, commenting on the 2019 attempt to enforce a nationally regulated waiting-time ceiling in ERs while continuing to decrease their funding

When I asked an expert triage nurse what it was like to work in the ER, he told me, "Eighty percent of the things we see here are not urgencies. We perform another kind of work than what we were trained for."

When speaking about the daily routine of the ER, both nurses and physicians distinguished between what it means in principle to work on the ward and what it is like in practice. Everyone I asked about the ER started by saying that the ER is a very dynamic place where "every day is different from the other, and you always learn something new."

They proceeded to add some version of "It's an experience that every health professional should have in their career," and "Here you are independent, take risks, face danger and work with various specialists." The work was saturated in adrenaline. It was quick and resolute. Patients in acute medical distress were stabilized. The rhetoric of war, as a fight against death and disease, was deeply entrenched in emergency care professionals' identities.

But there was another side to this image of heroic combat. When health care providers described what they actually did in the ER, their stories were quite distant from their heroic, romanticized image. They complained that the ER was full of people who should not really be there at all. They were "nonurgent" patients who came to the ER to seek help with complex chronic medical conditions and vulnerabilities, including those as diverse as diabetes, lack of housing, and mental health issues. Or they came to the ER with *cazzate* ("crap"—i.e., very low-priority cases that were the responsibility of their general practitioners [GPs]). Another type of individual whom health practitioners frequently encountered was *non funzionali* (meaning a person unable to cope with daily living, "not functioning," dysfunctional). These were people whom the ER staff deemed to have either psychological problems or were *casi sociali* (social work cases). The latter category grouped together lonely elderly people; individuals suffering from gender-related violence; and those who had migration, work, and family issues, precarious or no housing, alcohol and drug abuse problems, and/or economic instability.

All of these categories of people could be found in the ER. People who fell through the cracks of society came to the ER to seek the help and recognition that they felt was denied them elsewhere. Many were classified during triage as "nonurgent" patients, dubbed *utenti impropri*—"inappropriate users"—by the medical staff. These patients prompted many health care providers to realize that their instruments, training, and epistemological premises were, in a sense, inappropriate or inadequate to the task.

The presence of inappropriate users in the ER underscored the fact that the hospital did not just operate as a care provider. Inappropriate users foregrounded the fact that the ER was a core social institution that helped define the very experience of poverty and citizenship (Petryna and Follis 2015). Inappropriate users confronted the ER staff with stark evidence of social and economic injustices that, in the view of health care providers, largely fell outside the scope of their profession.

To face the flood of requests deemed nonurgent, many ERs in Italy have instituted backup fast-track services like a nurse's office, or *ambulatorio infermieristico*, licensed to "See and Treat" people's concerns immediately after triage assessment.[1] These services are usually located directly inside ERs. The nurse's office aims to deal with minor injuries, or other health issues that could easily be treated or redirected toward other public services by nurses, without making patients wait to be examined by a doctor. Other ERs have a GP's office inside the ER, open six to eight hours per day, dedicated to caring for people whose needs have been coded as white or green and who can be dealt with by simple treatments like painkillers, catheter changes, or medical prescriptions.[2] However, these makeshift solutions only slightly mitigate the structural gaps that Italians experience in accessing care, which they increasingly seek, as I have already noted, because they are aging and living under deteriorating socioeconomic conditions. People keep coming back to the ER, with their underlying needs unsolved and unattended to.

WHO IS INAPPROPRIATE?

"Signora, this is an inappropriate use of the *pronto soccorso* [ER]," a triage nurse named Monica said to signora Tania, an elderly woman of around seventy with long silver hair, after signora Tania told her that her foot had been hurting for more than a week. Adjusting her pink dress and speaking softly through the glass barrier of the ER reception desk, signora Tania explained that she had seen her GP but could not manage to wait ten days for an X-ray because her pain was unbearable. She simply "couldn't bear" (*sopportare*) the wait, she said, even though she had no detectable signs of trauma according to her GP.

Nurse Monica informed the signora that "this referral from your GP could have been used yesterday morning to go directly to the radiology ward to get an X-ray. Now the service is closed." Coming to the ER was inappropriate, since signora Tania could have dealt with her pain without coming to the ER or waiting another ten days.

Nurse Monica was informing signora Tania that a situation like hers did not belong in the ER not only because it did not fit the ER's definition of clinical urgency but also because in principle it was possible to address the problem elsewhere. For nonurgent cases, patients are expected to turn first to their GPs. That doctor may make a referral for an appointment for a diagnostic examination, social service support, a psychologist, a specialist consultation, or some other hospital's specific walk-in-service.

"If I had known that, I would have come yesterday," signora Tania said upon hearing this.

Nurse Monica glared and gesticulated to emphasize her explanation. "Because a pain in a foot for more than a week . . ." she said, attempting a conciliatory tone.

Signora Tania interrupted her, excusing herself by saying that she just had not known. "It has never happened to me before, so the GP did not explain anything to me," signora Tania explained.

"With a referral like this," continued Monica implacably, "you could have gone directly up to radiology. If you want, you can still go directly to radiology tomorrow."[3]

"No, I want to know what is wrong."

"Ok, *signora*, but I have to warn you: this is an inappropriate use of the ER. You are a white code and will have to wait for a long time."

ER staff like Nurse Monica understood inappropriate use only partly in relation to white codes, which, nationally, are estimated to compose around 24 percent of all ER patients.[4] The category of inappropriate users extends to encompass a great percentage of green codes (around 70% of patients) as well. Even though most health care providers judge green code cases to be a waste of their time, many are reticent to allocate a white code since, as we have seen, this means that the patient must pay a €25 "ticket" out-of-pocket "contact fee" plus a co-payment of €23 for each type of medical examination. A white code also condemns a person to spend as long as twelve hours waiting in the ER.

Signora Tania repeated that everything was her GP's fault and that she had tried using painkillers before she decided to come to the ER.

"You could have waited for the medical examination in ten days. Signora, there is no urgency," Nurse Monica repeated. After more than a week and without trauma of any sort, Nurse Monica judged signora Tania's situation to be nonurgent. It was unlikely to be a fracture, which would have fit the ER's clinical criteria of urgency. As Nurse Monica reflected later, it was clear that signora Tania's pain did not seem "unbearable" since she had managed to wait so long, and "surely" one could not do so with a "real" urgency. Such reasoning was a fairly common way for ER staff to make sense of suffering (cf. Johannessen 2019). Signora Tania, on the other hand, stressed a different understanding of pain—as something that affected her life in a negative embodied way, that impeded or hindered her daily activities and relations with others.

After signora Tania retreated from the glass wall to sit in the waiting room, Nurse Monica turned toward me and said, "At least, I've given her some health education" [*educazione sanitaria*]! She meant that she had given signora Tania instructions on how to become a "good service user" (*un buon utilizzatore del servizio*) to fit ER organizational demands.

Because it was an overcrowded Tuesday afternoon for the emergency service, signora Tania ended up waiting six hours to see the ER doctor.

THE PROPER FUNCTIONING OF THE *PRONTO SOCCORSO* DEPENDS UPON ALL OF US

Long waits like that endured by signora Tania were considered by the ER staff to be a kind of pedagogical resource. While they lamented such waits, and as noted above regarding the allocation of white codes (see also chapter 3), staff sometimes tried to shorten a wait by assigning a patient a more urgent code than they thought strictly necessary, many health care providers also regarded long waiting times as lessons designed to educate (*educare*) people on how to be good users (*un buon utente*). As Nurse Monica implied by talking about "health education," it was commonly thought that people like signora Tania needed to be taught how to "properly" use ER services. They needed to learn how to partake properly of the limited good offered at the ER and by the state through the hospital.

This same logic was apparent in an Italian government campaign, broadcast in 2012, to inform the population about how to use ERs correctly. This television campaign was notable partly for making the color-coding system I have been discussing explicit and partly for inviting viewers to understand the perspective of and even empathize with the triage nurses they would meet whenever they visited an ER. The commercial consisted of three vignettes of circus artists having accidents during a performance. For each vignette, a question appeared on the screen, encouraging viewers to judge the urgency of the accident.

The commercial begins with a drumroll and a shot of a bare-chested muscular man against a dark background, breathing fire from a torch. The first question pops up on the screen: "Is it a serious burn (red code) or heartburn (white code)" (Gravi ustioni [codice rosso] o bruciore di stomaco [codice bianco])? The next scene shows a contortionist in a turquoise leotard and high heels, who sneezes in a mid-stretch handstand position. Her back makes a loud cracking sound, but she pulls up her legs again, seemingly unharmed. The text reads: "Is it a fracture (green code) or a common cold (white code)" (Fattura [codice verde] o raffreddore [codice bianco])? Last comes a statuesque trapeze artist in a black leather leotard and dramatic makeup, swinging from a ring, flipping elegantly in the air and landing perfectly on the ground. At the end of her performance, a trapeze ring falls on her head. The question: "Is it a dangerous head trauma (yellow code) or a banal *cerchio alla testa* [literally, "ring to the head"]—i.e. headache (white code)?" While the three artists blur into the red circus tent in the background, the text on-screen is read by a reassuring male voice:

> Il buon funzionamento del Pronto Soccorso dipende da tutti noi.
> Impariamo come usarlo al meglio. Essere pronti aiuta il soccorso.[5]

> (The proper functioning of the ER depends on all of us. Let's learn how to use it best. Being ready [to properly use the ER] helps us help.)

This educational commercial focuses solely on fit athletic bodies whose possible medical problems signify interrupted health, not chronic conditions, aging, or social suffering. It uses humor to ask people to think twice about whether they really need to go to an ER when they have an accident or fall ill. It places the responsibility for this decision on the potential patients. It leaves the diagnosis up to them, and it implicitly condemns those who misidentify their symptoms as more serious than they are and who therefore ignorantly and selfishly clog up the "proper functioning of the ER." Structural issues such as troublesome access to primary care or long waits for specialists' examinations play no part here.

The commercial does not mention the increasing difficulty in reaching an overly busy GP, either by phone or in person. GPs also may not be able to solve many of the problems for which people ask for help without direct access to diagnostic or specialist consultations. People would have to be referred from the GP to a specialist for an appointment that may take weeks or even months. Even for dire conditions such as cancer, 6 percent of the Italian population in 2019 had to move between regions to access and be examined by a specialist (CENSIS 2023). Unable to move or pay for service in the growing private health care market, more than one Italian out of six in 2019 (12.2 million people) renounced accessing care altogether. Others, almost 50 percent of the Italian population in 2019, went directly to the ER.

The implicit take-home message of a commercial like this was that inappropriate users recklessly endanger the lives of those who are in the ER for legitimate urgent reasons. Illustrative of the neoliberal premise that a good society is primarily the responsibility not of the welfare state but of individual citizens, this government campaign encouraged a particular moral model of citizenship, one that ER staff at times invoked to enforce waiting as necessary. The commercial is illustrative of the state's selective governing of people's lives, a biopolitics that ignores people who cannot live up to its expectations (Foucault 1998, 136–139; 2004, 241–243).

Historically in the Italian context, this moral construction of what we may call "proper health citizenship"—that is, the individual's responsible use of state resources—immediately suggests its polar opposite: the *furbo*. This beloved Italian designation characterizes a person who is sly and dishonest but also clever and resourceful (Porter 2011; Molé 2013, 291). In contemporary Italy, an archetype of the *furbo* is former prime minister Silvio Berlusconi. The anthropologist Noelle Molé argues that Italians, in large measure through Berlusconi's well-publicized, excessive shenanigans and corruption, became both habituated to and disillusioned by irresponsible public behavior (Molé 2013, 292; Edwards 2005).

But the salience of the "furbo" in the Italian political debate, and discussion of the need for people to assume their role as a "good citizen," has also been instrumental, since the end of the 1960s, in depoliticizing and infantilizing working-class rebellions. Elio Petri's breathtaking film *Investigation over a Citizen above Any Suspicion* (*Indagine su un cittadino al di sopra di ogni sospetto*, 1970) showed how "immaturity," education, and "repression" were linked in the reasoning of state authorities during the political contestations against the Democrazia Cristiana, the Christian Democratic Party (in power since 1947 at the time of the film), between 1968 and 1973. In the role of a murderous, corrupt, high-ranking, right-wing police officer, who had been appointed with emergency powers to repress political turmoil, actor Gian Maria Volonté explains in an emphatic discourse: "People are children, the city is ill, others have the duty to heal or educate the people. We [the police] have to repress them! Repression is our vaccine. Repression is civilization!"[6]

In this cultural milieu, it is not surprising that in assigning signora Tania a white code, Nurse Monica told me that she wanted to make sure that the old woman was not "doing the *furba*" (*fare la furba*) and just coming to the ER in order to bypass normal hospital procedures and skip the queue. Nurse Monica was convinced she had acted in the best interests of both the organizational workflow of the ER and signora Tania, providing her with a lesson in being a good citizen.

The 2012 campaign discussed above was born out of the state's attempt to push responsibility for health care onto individuals in order to reduce the growing health care expenditures of the ER. For ER staff, though, something else was at stake in the division between appropriate and inappropriate demands for help. For them, what was under threat was their capacity to decide over urgency and to focus on what they considered to matter most. As in chapter 4, the balance between their medical authority and people's demands for care was increasingly fraught. The ER staff saw "education" as a way to reestablish order. They wanted to instill a particular moral idea of citizenship so that people who came to the ER for inappropriate reasons would think twice before doing it again. Education was a way of allowing triage to do its job.

This was what should have happened in theory.

In practice, though—even if a large number of the ER staff insisted on trying to provide the kind of education that Nurse Monica enunciated—the division between appropriate and inappropriate calls for help could not be enforced other than with waiting times. The bottom line was that, as nurses and doctors often repeated, "The ER's doors are always open" (Le porte del pronto soccorso sono sempre aperte). Sooner or later, everyone who arrives must be attended to.

No one was completely excluded from care in the ER, regardless of the urgency or the appropriateness of their demands. Such unconditional acceptance had a strong impact on how triage was carried out. It exposed triage as a vulnerable process of making a difference, one that people may drastically change by seeking attention in the ER for their emerging needs.

SOMETHING HAS CHANGED: THE ELDERLY, THE *CASI SOCIALI* (SOCIAL OUTCASTS), AND THE ANXIOUS

So why do people come to the ER even though, strictly speaking, they should not be there at all? The ER staff often offered stories about the consumer logic I discussed in chapter 4. "Oggi, tutti vogliono tutto e subito" (Nowadays, everyone wants it all and they want it now), they told me and one another.

"Oggi nessuno può aspettare" (Today, nobody can wait), Nurse Giovanni said in response to my question about overcrowding in the ER. "So people come to the ER to cut the line for normal medical appointments. Everybody is in much more of a hurry and society is much more rapid. Today, people order stuff on the web that arrives the next day at their homes. Why should they wait for health care?"

According to the ER staff, anxiety was a driving force that led people to the ER. Health care providers often nicknamed triage "the supermarket checkout" (*la cassa del supermercato*) to ironically portray their daily struggles with the attempts at line cutting and anxiety-driven "take-away" diagnostic tests, as discussed in chapter 4.

Together with anxiety, social abandonment was offered by the staff as an explanation for the presence of elderly people and *casi sociali* (social work cases) in the ER. "Families don't care for their children anymore, nor for their elderly relatives, who often die abandoned in hospital wards," Nurse Giovanni said. "We see more and more lonely elderly people and psychiatric cases among the youth here. These are the evils of the new millennium" (i mali del nuovo millennio).

This reflection echoed those of many health care providers I spoke to, and it prompted a question: What role does the ER play in the lives of people who are increasingly facing the hardship of aging, social abandonment, and existential anxiety?

Let us begin with the elderly. During 2018, 1.2 million people over the age of sixty-five in Italy—around 9 percent of the relevant population—defined themselves as isolated, with no contacts or few social contacts (CENSIS 2023). Lacking basic support, many elderly patients traveled constantly from nearby nursing homes to the ER for diagnostic examination and then back—only to start all over again a few days later (or even the same day) after they were hastily discharged.[7] Overall, 61 percent of ER visits in the Emilia-Romagna region were from patients over the age of sixty-five, despite that this population was only 23.9 percent of the region's total number of inhabitants (Osservatorio Nazionale 2018).

Elderly people in the ER were seen by staff as evidence that the ER was being inundated with low or nonurgent chronic illnesses, even though, at the same time, people over sixty-five received the majority of critical codes.[8] But elderly people kept coming back to the ER with unresolved issues. That was the case for signor Umberto and signora Flavia, whom I spoke to during a busy Christmas holiday night shift.

I sat down with the couple inside cubicle number three of the internal aisle of the triage area, where patients who needed to lie down were "parked" (*parcheggiati*), in ward jargon, while they waited to see the ER doctor. When I asked about their experience with the ER, signora Flavia said, "How much time do you have?"

"As long as you need," I answered.

Signora Flavia smiled. She took a deep breath and said, "Then let's start."

Signora Flavia, in her late seventies, looked with concern at her husband, signor Umberto, who was in his eighties. Signor Umberto was struggling to find a comfortable position on the stretcher. A drooping bag with a drip connected to his left kidney was leaking liquid from a surgically opened hole in his side. Signor Umberto appeared to be in rather intense pain.

In ER jargon, signor Umberto's situation was called "boarding time" (like other managerial jargon, the term, from English, was not translated into Italian). "Boarding time" referred to the increasingly common temporal discrepancy between the ER doctors' request for a hospital bed and access to one in an inner hospital ward. The 2008 financial crisis and the collapse of the right-wing coalition led by Silvio Berlusconi was followed by the unelected technical government of Mario Monti (composed of expert, nonpolitical, uncompromised members tasked with preventing state default).[9] It introduced the Decree Balduzzi (named after the minister of health) in 2012 to contain health care costs. One of the many egregious results of this decree was the further restriction of available hospital beds.

Signor Umberto had had a bed in the surgery ward. But due to bed shortages, he was discharged quickly. Lacking home assistance to manage catheter changes and painkillers, signor Umberto's kidney became infected again only two days after his latest surgery. He was back in the ER with an infection on "the very same day he was discharged from the hospital," signora Flavia exclaimed. "Why did they send him home right after the operation?" she asked me. "What should I do when he is in pain!? I bring him here!

"And this is not even the first time it has happened," she continued, working herself up. "As soon as you are discharged from the ward, they don't know who you are anymore. You feel like just a number, irrelevant. I have gone back and forth from the ER myself two times as well. Today, it is the third time in two weeks that we have come here to the ER!"

Signora Flavia listed a series of recurring waits due to chronic gallstones. All her health-seeking adventures were marked by marathon-like waits for specialists due to staff shortages and a lack of Italian National Health Service (NHS; Servizio Sanitario Nazionale) funding and the tangles of examinations and extreme difficulties in accessing the GP whom the NHS had assigned to her.

"Our doctor [GP] never makes home visits. He just gives us referrals to other specialists. We come to the ER to see a specialist in a reasonable amount of time. Umberto still has kidney stones, and I suffer from chronic gallstones," signora Flavia said. "We're always in the ER waiting for something."

People like signora Flavia and her husband are typical of the 66.7 percent of people over seventy years of age in Italy who have more than one chronic condition. Whenever I spoke to such people in the waiting room or the triage offices, they expressed despair at being invisible and disregarded during their frequent waits. Like signora Flavia and her husband, they seemed to be running in circles, waiting for different care services: their GP, hospital admissions and surgery, specialists and private practice appointments, and, when their medical conditions produced suffering they felt they could no longer bear, the ER.

In her conversation with me, signora Flavia remarked on the absence of fixed anchors in navigating the fragmented and underfinanced health care service. She complained about their GP, whom she and her husband mistrusted even though he was supposed to be their main reference point (*punto di riferimento*). In Italy today, GPs are increasingly few and overworked, each charged with the primary care of sometimes more than 1,500 patients. On average, over half of these patients are over sixty-five and have more than one chronic condition (Maciocco 2019). The current primary care system has ensured that GPs can be little more than *passa-carte*—that is, "paper pushers," mere bureaucrats whose role is to write out prescriptions and referrals to other specialists. Even getting to see a GP "can take weeks," signora Flavia reminded me.

In such a situation of uncertainty and continual waiting, the ER becomes an important anchor. Because it is not allowed to refuse care and because the waiting time to be seen by a doctor was measured in hours—not days, weeks or months—people like signora Flavia and her husband relied on the ER as the place to go to receive the care that they were unable to receive elsewhere.

The paradox—the tragedy—of this situation was that signora Flavia and signor Umberto, like so many others, were both dependent on and dissatisfied with the care provided by the ER because their needs could not possibly be met entirely by the ER itself. This was not so much due to resistance from or recalcitrance by the health care providers (even though, from the patients' point of view, the efforts by staff members such as nurse Monica to "educate" them might be taken that way) but to the fact that the ER was not intended or equipped to support chronic visits from patients with chronic medical conditions. To face the complex situation with which people like signora Flavia and her husband lived, ER staff could only improvise, tinkering with their limited means (e.g., changing catheters or bandages, injecting pain killers).

This impasse was not unique to elderly people who suffered from multiple chronic conditions. Another category of people who turned to the ER in times of need were so-called social outcasts (*casi sociali*) in search of the shelter and care denied them elsewhere.

THE "OUTCASTS" AND SOCIAL TRIAGE

"I used to smoke about thirty cigarettes a day. Now it depends on how many I find," said signor Sayd, a robust man of fifty-six who sat on a stretcher, wrapped in a scruffy trench coat. He was looking at his left worn-out shoe while Dr. Carmen, an experienced physician in her late thirties, wondered about his loud hacking cough. "And how long have you been living out on the street?" she asked.

Signor Sayd came to the ER after calling an ambulance for a pain in his chest. The rescue team found him in the city center, lying in a cardboard box behind a column to shield from the early January cold (between three and negative-three degrees Celsius), under a filthy brown-colored blanket. Now, like everything in his possession, the smelly blanket was stored under the stretcher in Dr. Carmen's office, put into the plastic bag that signor Sayd had insisted on bringing with him.

"A month and half," signor Sayd said after a pause, scratching his grayish beard. Dr. Carmen nodded and said, "You seem fine from the ECG. Now we will run blood tests and an X-ray to look at your strong cough."

"OK, signora. But, could you please also check this," signor Sayd said suddenly, pulling down his pants and pointing at the wide reddish stains on both his inner thighs extending to his pubis. His skin was dry and pockmarked by what looked like painful open crevices.

"I walk way too much," he said, while Dr. Carmen bent over to examine his groin. She explained that he had a bacterial infection and that he needed to wash the area more frequently to prevent further damage. Since this was impossible living on the street, Dr. Carmen prescribed him an antibacterial cream to use twice a day. Then she sent him to get his X-ray for the cough.

I escorted signor Sayd to the radiology room. While waiting for the results of his X-ray, we chatted. And like so many patients who seemed to welcome the chance to talk, he began to tell me his life history.

"I come from a little village in Morocco," he began. "I went to France in 1987, and at twenty-four, I was studying physics in Paris. I wanted to become a nuclear physicist. I had a scholarship back then, like you do," he said, referring to my explanation that I was a graduate student studying in Sweden.

"I hope it will turn out for the better for you," he said laconically. "I left everything for a woman.

"I came to Italy with her but she dumped me soon after. I stayed in Lombardy [a region in the north of Italy] for a while, where my Moroccan friends lived. We started selling things on the street. We got good at it, and we began selling dresses and other stuff. Then, I moved to Emilia-Romagna and worked as a construction worker and carpenter. I've done that since the end of the nineties. But since 2010, things have become more difficult."

Signor Sayd was referring to the housing market collapse in Italy from 2008 when, because of the global financial crisis, bank loans became widely inaccessible, and many houses remained unsold. The construction business was hit hard.

"All the construction sites I was working for shut down, one after another. And after the earthquake, many other enterprises went bankrupt."

Signor Sayd let his voice sink to a grave tone as he remembered the disastrous effects of the 6.1 magnitude earthquake that struck the Emilia-Romagna region in 2012. The quake resulted in 27 deaths, 300 people injured, 15,000 evacuated from their homes, and damage amounting to more than €13 million.

"I started drinking and smoking, things I had never done before," he said, in between coughs. "A social worker helped me out as well as she could. But I am not an asylum seeker, and my papers are all in order. That meant that I could not access housing reserved for people waiting for their papers. But at least I'm not as badly off as people who are refused asylum. They don't get anything at all. Here in Italy, no one cares for people on the streets. The police don't take you to a dormitory, and the social services don't exist. In France and Germany, things are better. I might go there sometime soon."

Not wanting to live on the street but unable to obtain assistance anywhere else, signor Sayd turned to Emergenza Freddo (Cold Emergency), a national crisis program that aimed to provide beds in public dormitories during wintertime to prevent people from sleeping outdoors (and risking death) in the cold. But signor Sayd was unsuccessful there too.

Feeling depressed, sick, and cold and rebuffed by the Italian welfare state, signor Sayd's last hope was the ER. Like signora Flavia and her husband, who frequently came to the ER not to resolve a medical emergency but as a way to deal with the tangled and lethargic state of the Italian health care system, signor

Sayd turned to the ER not primarily to resolve an urgent medical condition but rather as a way of coping with his deteriorating housing situation and to receive some kind of recognition as a human being. But as with signora Flavia and her husband, the ER could only provide makeshift solutions in which improvisation played a key role.

This improvisation was evident in what happened when I escorted signor Sayd back to cubicle number five in the internal triage aisle. I was pulling the white curtains to give him some privacy when Dr. Carmen joined us, holding the X-ray results. "What shall we do?" she said. "You have liquid in your lungs. You cannot go back outside. But there are no beds available right now."

Seemingly having foreseen this outcome, signor Sayd asked for a medical certificate that would grant him a spot in the communal dormitory as a protected hospital discharge (*dimissione protetta*) in the Emergenza Freddo program. Dr. Carmen agreed to this, adding, "Rest here for the moment. In the morning I will call the dormitory myself to make sure they will accept you there."

Grateful, signor Sayd went to sleep on the stretcher in cubicle number five. I saw signor Sayd return to the ER multiple times to find shelter or basic (and thus, in principle, inappropriate) medical assistance. He was not alone. In 2018, five million people (8.9% of the Italian population) were living below the threshold of absolute poverty, defined as a state in which the subject lacks the means to meet their basic needs (e.g., food, water, shelter, basic education, and health care; Schweiger 2020). Many of these people, having lost their housing, were not entitled to be registered with a GP because they lacked a fixed address. As signor Sayd noted, such a situation had an especially hard impact on migrants, who, due to increasingly draconian "border security" laws enacted from 2002, had restricted access to health care and work permits (Riccio 2007, 26–36; cf. Fassin 2005, in France).[10] Many such individuals, both migrants and Italian nationals, came to the ER at some point or another with chest pains or headaches, knowing that they would be examined. During their wait, they could warm themselves or, if they were lucky enough, be invited to recline on a stretcher, temporarily relieved of the fatigue of life on the street.

ANXIETY AND WORK PRECARITY

In his work on the HIV outbreak of the 1990s in West Africa, the anthropologist Vinh-Kim Nguyen (2010, 180–183) describes how multiple forms of triage can intersect in people's search for better life chances. Nguyen details different kinds of social and medical triage that, throughout the colonial and contemporary history of Côte d'Ivoire, shaped biopower (in the sense of the "marshaling of vital forces" of the population) through the "exercise of power over life" by the French colonial authorities first and later by international humanitarian aid programs (Nguyen 2010, 111–136).

In a similar fashion, people like signora Flavia and her husband and signor Sayd are impacted by societal processes of exclusion, and partly for this reason, they resort to the ER as a means of dealing with social abandonment. Contrary to what Nguyen highlights, though, people's makeshift use of state aid—the ER in this case—did not create a parallel structure to state authority (2010, 175–183). Individuals like signora Flavia and signor Sayd did not self-organize like the local nongovernmental organizations and HIV-positive patients' self-aid groups that Nguyen describes (2010, 89–110). The recurring demands of people like signora Flavia and signor Sayd did not create a kind of parallel triage. But they nevertheless directly influenced the ER.

They did this by compelling a process of selection that insisted on a momentary solution—like providing a Band-Aid, perhaps—to people's broader conditions of health and existential precarity. Triage in the ER still created temporary distinctions such as the color codes, corresponding to different waiting times. But those boundaries, under pressure by people who returned multiple times, were permeable. Patients could receive different color codes, and sooner or later, everyone was attended to. Triage assumed a recursive, cyclical structure, one that evolved along people's recurring attempts to access makeshift means of care, which never completely failed but which frequently was not entirely successful either.

In addition to elderly people and people like signor Sayed who found himself living on the street, many young and middle-aged people were driven to the ER by precarious working conditions to access care that was deemed by the staff as not urgent.

Precarity looms large in the anthropological literature about Italy, where it is linked to people's diminishing economic support and worsening working conditions and to increasing "dispossession" from the possibility of planning ahead and having a stable, secure future. "Precarity" here denotes an existential condition that lacks the material means—be they socioeconomic or medical—to feel secure and stable (Allison 2012, 2013; Tsing 2015). The word is a "shorthand [to] document the multiple forms of nightmarish dispossession and injury" that our times entail and for which people seek urgent help in the ER (Muehlebach 2013).

Without paid sick leave and unable to go to a GP due to their limited office hours (on average, three hours a day, five days a week),[11] people who worked as interns or under temporary contracts came to the ER to cope with stress and deteriorating physical and mental health. Work precarity materialized in the ER as an embodied sense of inadequacy, instilled by the pressing demands of the relatively newly shaped Italian neoliberal job market.

Since 2003, after the Legge Biagi (the Biagi Law, named after Mario Biagi, a consultant with the Ministry of Welfare), which introduced new kinds of job contracts with fewer rights for workers, the conditions of employment in Italy were dramatically restructured. From having been a highly *tutelato* (safeguarded)

Fordist system based on non–fixed-term contracts (*contratti a tempo indetermi-nato*) for employees, conditions shifted to a neoliberal labor market (such as those of the United States and United Kingdom) based mostly on *contratti prec-ari* (precarious—i.e., fixed-term—contracts, usually short-term and with no or limited worker protection or welfare benefits; Porcellana 2022). The dream of lifelong employment, which had animated the hopes of generations since the 1960s economic boom, began to come to nothing. The "Jobs Act," a 2014 labor reform, further expanded the social and economic split between long-term and short-term workers of a "two-tier workforce" (Molé 2011, 8–10). The fact that the Jobs Act was given an English name instead of a corresponding Italian name (such as something like Azione del Lavoro) was a nod to the futuristic aim of the reform and also a tip of the hat to an established cultural script that saw the United States and United Kingdom as more advanced and modern than Italy.

This act ascribed Fordist models of production to the past. Such models saw it as entrepreneurs' duty to provide workers with welfare that both secured fam-ilies' financial stability and their role as consumers in what was a booming capi-tal market between the 1960s and the early 1990s (Muehlebach 2013). Back then, lifelong employment was also a way for the Christian Democratic Party to govern the aspiration of the population. Providing people with economic secu-rity, the party asked for votes in return. Flexibility and insecurity—the social evils that the Christian Democratic Party tried to avoid—were instead ascribed by the Jobs Act to a new supposedly prosperous neoliberal future.

In 2018, *i precari* (the precariat) became a category consisting of almost four million people in Italy, mostly under the age of forty or older independent work-ers who were left alone to deal with economic stagnation. The anthropologist Noelle Molé (2012) has discussed the "haunting of solidarity in post-Fordist Italy" as the longing for the bygone social and work security in a cultural setting where unemployment was regarded as "social death" (Molé 2012, 384–391; Capello 2020). More often subject to emotional and physical harassment at work (referred to—again, tellingly—by the English word "mobbing" in Italy) and unable to plan ahead for their future, many *precari*—that is, people who have fallen victim to being "precarious"—became subject to ever-greater social and economic insecurity. Feeling inadequate, people increasingly turned to medical diagnoses to actively try to renegotiate the space they inhabited as precarious workers having to live up to social expectations still grounded in bygone illu-sions of Fordist security.

In the work by the anthropologist Vinh-Kim Nguyen mentioned above, a similar process of "self-fashioning" is described, in which HIV-positive young people in Côte d'Ivoire invested time and resources in practicing bodybuilding. The young people Nguyen discusses dreamed of becoming bodyguards in the French security industry. They self-fashioned to fit a kind of personhood that, in addition to providing them with employment, would also grant them access to antiretroviral therapies (Nguyen 2010, 152–154). In a context of colonial global inequity, "self-fashioning was a powerful tool for confronting economic uncertainty and keeping alive ideas of progress and good life" (Nguyen 2010, 150).

In the ER, this tendency was exemplified by Valentina (who asked me not to call her *signora*), a thirty-year-old woman who arrived at the ER directly from work. Valentina told me that she was struggling to affirm herself as a "real" attorney in an important local law firm. Officially, she was in the last year of her internship as a trainee attorney, but her boss and co-workers mostly treated her as a secretary, belittling her professional skills. She had begun to suffer from abdominal and back pain. Her GP had very limited office hours, while Valentina worked sometimes twelve hours a day. Unable to access her GP, Valentina started coming frequently to the ER to obtain painkillers and for in-depth diagnostic evaluations. Because she did not have either the time to go to her GP or the money to be referred to private practice, Valentina could only keep coming back to the ER to access medical examinations. Time after time, different ER examinations gradually constructed a fragmented diagnostic picture without continuity of care. She told me that she had also recently developed migraines, and her co-workers had started to suspect that her abdominal and back pains were a way to obtain sick leave to which, according to the terms of her employment contract, she was not entitled. Her precarious employment, and hence, financial situation, made her panic. Her partner was depressed and unemployed, and the couple were living on her limited salary. Valentina told me that she felt trapped.

Longing to become a mother, Valentina and her partner had been trying unsuccessfully to conceive for two years. She had paid for all sorts of medical tests to identify fertility issues, but nothing had come up. Her partner, on the other hand, had refused to submit to a fertility test. The couple had been bickering frequently lately, and Valentina's pains in her abdomen had increased.

Defining what was happening in her abdomen was vital to Valentina; the pain was central to everything that was happening in her life. She blamed her suffering for not being able to live up to the expectations of her boss and co-workers. It was also the cause, she felt, of her inability to conceive and of the increasingly unsatisfying relationship with her partner.

Like others trying to cope with symptoms related to their precarious working conditions and lack of access to their GPs or being unable to deal with the long waiting time for specialists' consultations, Valentina came back to the ER many times to find out, she told me, "what is wrong with me." Anxiety and suffering stemming from dealing with broader social forces constituted a different kind of urgency for the isolated elderly, for the social outcasts or the homeless, and for the *precari* feeling on the verge of a social death.

PRIVATIZATION: WHO CAN AFFORD CARE?

The different kinds of people who sought help from the ER for reasons the staff deemed nonurgent seemed to have something in common. Elderly people suffering from multiple chronic conditions came frequently to the ER in search of some sort of anchor in the context of their social abandonment. The *casi sociali* (social work cases) sometimes turned to the ER to cope with harsh living conditions. Last, so-called anxious people (*gli ansiosi*) came to the ER in an attempt to try to make sense of a life that seemed buffeted by social and economic forces far beyond their comprehension or control. One feature of contemporary society crosscuts the situations of all these inappropriate users.

That feature is the market.

The very distinction between "proper" and "inappropriate" users implies a link between public health and private enterprises. The term "user" (*utente*) equates patients with service-oriented "customers/clients" and foregrounds independent choice (Mol 2008, 25–26). The emphasis on individual responsibility in care seeking both obscures structural hindrances to obtaining health care and allows the state to blame patients and charge them with contact fees (the *ticket*), which are applied to specialist examinations.[12]

Other terms exist that provide a different framing of responsibility, one that foregrounds structural failures in addressing people's needs. For instance, in Germany people seeking help for issues judged as not urgent by medical staff are called "wrongly guided patients" or "misguided patients" (Ger. *fehlgeleitete Patienten*). The German label implies that the patients have been misled or provided with incorrect information by the relevant authorities. It suggests more of a misunderstanding than active deception, being *furbo*, and line cutting, which is emphasized by the terms commonly used in public health care systems that have been heavily affected by processes of privatization, such as the Italian *untenti impropri* or the UK inappropriate users.

According to the medical historian Giorgio Cosmacini (2016, 546–561), a cultural shift occurred in Italy in the 1990s with the national reorganizing decree 502 of 1992 that turned local health units (*unità di salute locale*) into *aziende* (meaning private enterprises, *azienda sanitaria locale*). The decree entrusted more administrative functions to health care providers within the Italian NHS. But such new administrative functions were explicitly centered around the task of containing costs and cutting health care budgets. As a result, health care professionals saw their paperwork double and their financial resources drastically reduce.

Discourses about efficiency multiplied in health care simultaneously with guidelines intended to sideline professionals' individual judgment discretion and foster the standardization of medical practice. The *aziendalizzazione* (the process of becoming an *azienda*—i.e., enterprise) focused on rationalization and performance efficiency and thereby enabled a closer collaboration with private interests. Since the 1990s, private health care facilities have increasingly started taking over services that previously had been offered by the public health service.

A case in point is offered by the ER itself. The outsourcing of emergency services started to appear as a consequence of the introduction of the DRG financial system (1994). As we saw in chapter 4, the DRG system—working according to the principle that the more diagnoses a hospital made, the more a hospital administration could profit from regional funds—excluded the ER that faced increasing expenses due to overcrowding. Unable to afford new personnel, ERs outsourced contracts to private companies in order to hire short-term staff, often for just a few months. Though they are not granted any social security benefits, the compensation of physicians and nurses under private contracts is sometimes more than double the salary of the staff hired in the public system. This further eroded public services' capacity to retain a workforce, and a hiring freeze was imposed in 2012.

Even though particularly dire, the situation of ERs is not unique. Unable to hire new staff to cover the delivery of care that people increasingly require, the public system has been outsourcing medical services at an increasing pace.

As public capital started flowing into private enterprises, those private health care options widened their influence and scope. One result of this is that many extremely popular diagnostic and specialist examinations, such as X-rays, CAT scans, and MRI scans,[13] which generally have long waiting times in public facilities, have become targeted by private practices, who present their services as the solution to the "problem" of public health care.

In addition to offering quicker diagnostic examinations, private health care was also supported by a 1999 law that allowed both what is known as *intramoenia* (private practice allowance inside public hospitals) and *extramoenia* (private practice allowance outside public hospitals). This law allowed physicians who worked in public facilities to also work in private practice. Some of the patients I spoke to told me that it was not rare to be told by a specialist working in a public hospital that they could either wait three or more months for a consultation or pay an out-of-pocket fee of anywhere from €90 to €300, or more, and receive the consultation immediately *by the same doctor working in the same public health care facility* but in a private capacity.

The flow of public capital, professionals, and resources into the private market was accompanied by a systemic definancing of the NHS, particularly after the economic crisis of 2008. As noted in chapter 1, from 2010 to 2019 funding to public health care was cut by €37 billion. By portraying the NHS as incapable of maintaining its universal coverage due to growing financial costs, defunding was disguised. Austerity measures and the lobbying of private interests in health marketization, such as private insurance companies, were all effectively hidden from public discourse.

A report on health expenditures in Italy from 2019 showed that almost one person out of two (19.6 million people, 44% of the Italian population) had paid out-of-pocket fees for private health services, for a total expenditure of €37.7 billion (7.2% more since 2014).[14] This trend was explained by the shortcomings of an increasingly underfinanced public health service, a health care service that in 35.8 percent of cases was unable to cover even the basic care rights of the population due to its increasingly long waits for specialist consultations or exams (basic level of assistance [*livelli essenziali di assistenza*]).

TRIAGE AT AN IMPASSE

The increasing gap between those who can afford to turn to the private system and those who only have access to the heavily underfinanced public health system (Costa et al. 2016) put triage in the ER in a situation of impasse. Regardless of whether they are regarded by staff as inappropriate users or not, for many people the ER is the only option to access in-depth diagnostic tools and care delivered in what people consider to be a reasonable amount of time

This dynamic has had a significant impact on triage itself, turning it from a singular moment of selection, of decision over urgency, into a kind of cyclic process that deals with people who return to the ER multiple times to negotiate makeshift care solutions for their health issues. The solutions they are offered are almost inevitably short term and inadequate because the ER is not designed to sustain the long-term care that people are increasingly demanding.

Because it can neither refuse care nor completely support people's situations of precarity and abandonment, triage is at an impasse in the ER. This impasse entails a shift from a singularity of selection to a longue durée of repetition. It turns what formerly was a singular moment of making a difference into a recursive cycle of demands and inconclusive solutions in which differences cannot be held stable. The circular movement of triage develops into a more general change in the governance of care given by the impossibility of state governmentality to be fully enforced. This impossibility creates a paradox in which new spaces of care and improvisation are possible, and a new way to understand urgency could emerge.

Indeed, the cycle of triage at an impasse did not only adversely affect the rapid pacing of temporality that was considered by all the ER staff with whom I spoke as characterizing their work. It was also productive of new relations in the ER that had practical consequences for patients, health professionals, and state health care governance.

First, as people facing harsh living conditions and debilitating structural forces bring their concerns to the ER, clinical urgency is not the only thing at stake in care negotiations. People's overcrowding of the ER turned neoliberal governance of care on its tail. It forced the Italian state to address needs that the market-driven policies I described above intentionally attempted to ignore. For many so-called inappropriate users, visiting the ER was the only way to obtain a sort of "second-class" health citizenship—in other words, a precarious membership and possibility of negotiating an active role in society (Porter 2011; Petryna 2013; Petryna and Follis 2015). It was precarious because, contrary to the "proper health citizenship" that people who could pay for private health services could afford, a second-class health citizenship was created by the unstable, improvised solutions negotiated recursively in the ER by patients.[15] Not having anywhere else to go, inappropriate users attempted to increase their odds of coping with life in worsening social and economic conditions by seeking some form of control over their deteriorating bodily conditions.

Second, the recurrence of demands for help from patients who kept returning to the ER has become the basis for a new economy of attention. ER staff have realized that they need to pay more attention to how patients live in the world and what kinds of problems they face there. The engulfment of triage in ERs across the country demonstrates how a change in the microeconomy of attention in the ward can alter the macroeconomy of attention, which articulates the way the Italian state manages the life of its citizens and its biopolitics.

But recurring visits did not just change the nature of the economy of attention in the ER; they also changed its tenor. The cyclic structure of demands for help produced an economy of attention increasingly centered around conflict, as fatigue and frustration on both sides set in and took root.

The ER has become a place of friction. Partly to deal with this tension, "inappropriateness" was developed as a defensive mechanism to shield what the staff envisioned as the ER's mission from precisely the kinds of phenomena that increasingly drove patients to seek it. The difference between appropriate and inappropriate in the ER was carved out of an assemblage of set organizational rules, workflow habits, available means, moral imperatives, and care ethics connected both to professional identity and to what it meant for the ER staff to be "emergency workers," getting their work done on their own terms.

In addressing so-called inappropriate users, health care providers also had to become creative. Care negotiations oscillated between frustration toward inappropriate use, as in the example of Nurse Monica and the woman with the hurt foot, and sincere attempts to acknowledge patients' situations and support their capacity to remain healthy, as Dr. Carmen did by calling the dormitory to make sure signor Sayd would receive a warm place to sleep.

In a discussion about the range of patients that come to the ER for assistance, a doctor once told me that "in the end, maybe even in a subliminal way, the patient just wants to understand what's going on, putting some order to all the stuff she has done over weeks, months, and even years." This recognition of the complexity of care was mirrored in another interview, this one in the waiting room, with a man around sixty who had just been labeled a white code after triage.

Talking about his persistent cough, he told me how after having seen his wife slowly pass away from lung cancer, he could not help being scared of his own coughing, especially since it had recurred intermittently during the previous two years. Reflecting on being given a white code, he told me that he had been coming back and forth from the ER as he unfortunately could not access his GP due to the limited office hours and could not afford to turn to private practice. Even though he told me he understood why he had been given a white code after triage, he wondered what else he could have done. He did not blame the ER staff for his waiting but wondered how he could get the basic care he needed without referring to the ER.

When I told him that he was not alone in facing such a situation of impasse, he coughed, nodded, and said quietly: "It is important that *they* [I assume the state, the government, the hospital administration, the powers that be] look into this situation more closely. Because people don't know what the f-ck to do (*cosa cazzo fare*)."

6 · MISTRUST IN THE ER

Fidarsi è bene, non fidarsi è meglio.
(To trust is good, not to trust is better.)

—Italian proverb

The defunding of medical care by the Italian government and the increasing impoverishment of the population has resulted in various structural and temporal changes, as detailed in chapter 5. But it has also contributed to a change in sensibility or mood. ER staff often told me that "things have changed" (le cose sono cambiate) and that they felt that communication with patients was becoming increasingly difficult. "People no longer trust us to make decisions," an experienced physician remarked at the end of a tiring night shift. "They mistrust the entire health system."[1]

Litigation, often born of mistrust, has increased dramatically in the ER. As notoriously in the United States, patients in Italy can directly sue a health professional for malpractice.[2] And they do: patients and their families are suing hospitals and individual doctors and nurses at unprecedented rates, for malpractice (malasanità [bad health care]), being rude, or denying them medication or a bed in the hospital to more serious gross negligence or culpability (colpa grave o gravissima) that resulted in death. Between 2004 and 2019, there was one lawsuit for malpractice every ten days for each public health care structure nationally. The leading area for a malpractice lawsuit is surgery (38.5% of all lawsuits). ERs attract 12.6 percent of all lawsuits, with steady increases each year.[3] A similar increase also happened during the first two years of the pandemic, when requests for refunds climbed up to an average of €127,000.

Law firms that began flourishing in the late 1990s exhorted patients to pursue lawsuits, claiming on billboards and on local television commercials that people "deserved" compensation (vi meritate un rimborso). Hospital staff felt vulnerable. They told me that they could count on little support from hospital administration in the face of a lawsuit from a dissatisfied patient, as exemplified by Dr. Paolo's confrontation with signora Gianna (chapter 4). They joked morosely that the hospital's motto had become "Keep Customers Happy" (Fare felice il cliente). Nurses and doctors were increasingly concerned that they should write down everything they did, as they became aware that the basis for their medical decisions could be contested by patients and used against them in court.

One result of this anxiety was that nurses and doctors spent a great amount of their already limited time bent over their computer keyboards, filling in forms, documenting in detail everything they did. Their concern with detail, and the bureaucratic systems in place to ensure this, was a way of dealing with both the possibility of litigation and the hospital's increased emphasis on an audit culture based on "rationalization"—that is, cost reduction (Strathern 2000; Kipnis 2008; Hull 2012, 629–630).

The mistrust that health care practitioners experienced from patients was reciprocal. Practitioners routinely mistrusted many of the patients they saw. ER staff constantly suspected people of "doing the *furba*" and attempting to skip long waiting lines for specialists' consultations or in-depth diagnostic examination in a hospital ward. Health care providers often questioned, openly or silently, the reasons why people came to the ER, as we saw in the cases of signora Gianna, in chapter 4, and signora Tania, in chapter 5. To evaluate those reasons, practitioners cross-referenced patients' accounts with the documents that they could access in the hospital-specific computer database. Health care practitioners also increasingly preferred to base their assessment of a patient's state on bodily signs rather than the patient's account of suffering (cf. Ticktin 2011). Health care providers were suspicious and even dismissive when patients reported suffering without obvious medical signs.

So mistrust in the ER was mutual, and importantly, it structured interactions. Those interactions affected how the negotiation of urgency unfolded.

TRIAGE AND THE NEGLECTED OPPOSITE OF TRUST

The erosion of trust in state institutions such as hospitals is not a uniquely Italian phenomenon. According to public health scholar David Shore (2006, 3, 215–225), trust in the state and health care authorities in both high- and middle-income settings was even then in crisis, "compromising medical outcomes [and] endangering patients' lives and wellbeing." Shore focused on the United States and its health system, and he listed the reasons why trust is in crisis. One was the pervasiveness of for-profit health care, in which businesses were more concerned with capital gains than patients' actual care and outcomes (Shore 2006, 7–14). Another reason was the skyrocketing costs of health care due to the lengthening of life expectancy and the increasing presence of expensive medical technologies. Such changes in health care demand and delivery resulted in decreasing quality of care delivered to patients when hospitals and insurance companies tried to contain health care costs (Shore 2006, 49–76; cf. Napier et al. 2014).

Other research on hospital health care delivery shows similar patterns. For instance, in examining diverse hospital settings in both the United States and

Europe, the bioethicist Nancy Berlinger (2016, 112–126, 193) explains how institutional constraints such as stringent protocols limit the time to speak with and examine patients and how the excess of bureaucracy sometimes makes it impossible for practitioners to help their patients, contributing to a spiraling lack of care and trust (see also Chambliss 1996). The public health scholar Lucy Gilson (2006) points out that health professionals' lack of training in communication skills produces flaws in their capacity to build trust. The anthropologists Arthur Kleinman and Sjaak van der Geest (2009, 162–163) suggest that trust is undermined by biomedicine's intense focus on the technical aspects of medicine, at the expense of its caregiving dimensions, which are more emotionally involved and morally driven. These larger studies were conducted a decade or more ago; the factors contributing to the lack of trust have only increased since then.

These research articles focus on trust. But mistrust—and its effects in relation to care access and delivery—is just as important to understand and is an understudied topic. As the anthropologist Florian Mühlfried (2019) recently observed, there are numerous studies on trust in political science, philosophy, sociology, and public health studies, but this research tends to treat mistrust as an absence—as a lack or a crisis of trust—rather than as a force in its own right.[4] The tendency to address mistrust as a lack of trust is particularly clear in research in public health publications, like the work by Shore (2006), who lists motives for which trust is in crisis and how it might be won back by policy-makers and health care workers.

Mistrust has been addressed by anthropologists working on triage and governmentality.[5] Studies of triage in anthropology focus on how people's requests for help are assessed by health professionals—or other state or humanitarian aid workers—as either trustworthy or untrustworthy in reference to diverse medical and bureaucratic procedures. The anthropologist Miriam Ticktin (2011), for instance, explored how in 2007, French state authorities started to base decisions about migrants' asylum seeking on biological signs because they mistrusted people's narrative accounts of their suffering. Another example is the anthropologist Adriana Petryna's research (2013) on how Ukrainian citizens' claims for disability pensions after the Chernobyl nuclear disaster raised suspicion among health care experts and bureaucratic state apparatuses. While valuable for demonstrating the various ways in which people are granted or denied, say, political asylum or welfare benefits, work like Ticktin's and Petryna's does not directly identify mistrust as a relational resource. Rather, mistrust remains in the background of this richly theorized work. Mistrust as a relational, interactional resource, however, is what we clearly see in the ER.

Matthew Carey (2017, 1–14) has challenged the view of mistrust as equivalent to a lack of trust and instead sees mistrust as an attitude with its own social forms, ones that develop differently from the orientations based on trust. Working with people living in the Atlas Mountains of Morocco and arguing against an essentialist view of trust as something necessarily good, Carey argues that mistrust does not necessarily undermine sociality. Instead, mistrust may become a nexus of sociality, enabling productive ways of interacting with others.

Suspicion, lying, and deception as manifestations of mistrust may be ways of constructing others as essentially unknowable, "expected to lapse and sometimes fail: to betray their friends, break their word, and let people down" (Carey 2017, 40). Such an orientation may facilitate the granting of forgiveness more easily, Carey argues, and contribute to building up a tolerant environment that fosters social cohesion and individual reinvention. The people he worked with rarely committed to a serious search for truth, and apparently none felt social pressure to be evaluated, or to evaluate others, as trustworthy or predictable (Carey 2017, 23–25, 40–45).

Mühlfried (2019) has also explored the practical effects of mistrust. Drawing on ethnographic examples from Eastern Europe and the country of Georgia, Mühlfried provides an analytics of mistrust by looking at its kaleidoscopic effects—its capacity to facilitate assessments of other people's intentions, to avoid direct conflicts, as a way of dealing with strangers, or as a way of coping with precarious situations of resource shortages or political disorder (2019, 33–47, 90–91; see also Mühlfried 2017).

Following these authors, I consider mistrust in the ER as an interactional resource that is rarely articulated explicitly. It manifests as lying, deception, avoidance, double agendas, doubt, and suspicion. For instance, patients in the ER sometimes decided to dramatize details they assumed might be relevant (e.g., pregnancy) or omit those they suspected might not be relevant or which might result in judgment (e.g., drug use), with the goal of having their health needs met to their satisfaction. Doctors and nurses at times withheld information or expressed themselves ambiguously, in order to better manage people's reactions and their long waiting times. Duplicity, and the mistrust that both gave rise to and resulted from it, suffused the ER.

Such relations of mistrust, however, frequently facilitated rather than reduced complexity. Mistrust created a space where different perspectives on care could coexist. Such space was key within a governance of care that, as we have seen, was increasingly fraught with conflict.

Both a destructive and productive force in the ER, mistrust manifested differently according to power relations and interaction dynamics at play. Four vectors of mistrust coexisted in the interactional space of the ER. First, health care providers mistrusted patients' accounts. Second, mistrust was sometimes mutual between health care providers and patients. And third, patients and the people who accompanied them to the ER could mistrust the health care providers' diagnosis and advice. A fourth vector of mistrust also obviously existed: mistrust between health care providers themselves. We saw an example of this in chapter 4 when Dr. Paolo told me that he mistrusted his colleagues to "have the guts" to openly support him in his dispute with signora Gianna. Even though this type of mistrust affected the way in which urgency came into being in the ER, I do not thematize it here because it is only indirectly relevant to my concern with unraveling the economy of attention that created urgency in the ER. I address mistrust between health care providers when it is directly relevant to the interactions I analyze, such as the conflict between Dr. Paolo and signora Gianna.

DAILY ENCOUNTERS WITH MISTRUST IN TRIAGE

In all of its shapes and dynamics, mistrust stood in a mutually constitutive relationship with trust. Rather like urgency and waiting, mistrust and trust coexisted in different but complementary relations in the daily practice of triage.

In a context marked by the uncertainties of understaffing and overcrowding, one thing was all too certain in the ER to both staff and patients: the activities that occurred in the ER were inherently unpredictable. No one could tell when the emergency phone would ring. No one could foresee car crashes, heart attacks, or the abrupt reactions of the people waiting: yelling, crying desperately, threatening each other, or acting violently toward health care providers. No one could predict when an overworked nurse or doctor would simply have had enough and react or end up feeling burned-out, exhausted by the increasingly demanding work shifts and insufficient rest. Unfolding primarily among people who were strangers to each other, negotiations of urgency in the ER constantly shifted focus, resources, and waiting time in unforeseeable ways.

Mistrust was key in dealing with unpredictability, and on the ward, mistrust took many shapes. For instance, once the infusions contained in intravenous vials were empty, many patients nervously asked nurses to turn off their drips because they were afraid that a bubble of air could find its way inside their veins and potentially kill them. "If that could really happen," I once heard a nurse patiently explaining to a man who had anxiously requested that his drip be turned off, "we would shut the drip off immediately." The man shrugged his shoulders while the nurse turned off his drip. ER staff sometimes became frustrated with people whose entire knowledge of human bodies and medical care seemed to be gleaned from American television shows, where murderous air bubbles figure prominently.

Sensationalistic media reporting on malpractice cases also invited patients to be suspicious of medical staff. An extreme example, embedded in the Italian consciousness because of relentless reporting, was the 2014 case of the "killer nurse" (*infermiera killer*) in Lugo, a small city in Emilia-Romagna. Police investigators described the nurse as "manipulative" and "disturbingly merciless."[6] She took pictures of herself mocking the corpse of her victim, a seriously ill seventy-eight-year-old woman, whom she had injected with a fatal dose of potassium. These photos and the resulting outrage went viral on all media platforms. Another case that garnered national attention was one in the northern city of Bolzano, in which a nurse mistakenly injected a man in a nursing home with a drug that ended up killing him.[7] Many patients would also have heard about the reported cases of infections after surgery due to bandages and surgical tools being forgotten in patients' abdomens.[8] The Italian Institute for Monitoring Insurance Activities (Istituto Italiano di Vigilanza Sulle Assicurazioni [IVASS]) reported 17,000 medical errors in the public health care system in 2018 alone.[9] Unsurprisingly, the annual increase of documented medical errors (up 3% between 2017 and 2018) went hand in hand with the progressive underfinancing of the public health system.

Mistrust became particularly visible when dealing with situations of great uncertainty. During a busy afternoon in the ER, when crowding in the external waiting room was intense, signora Emma, a woman of about eighty, arrived in an ambulance. After conducting a brief evaluation of her condition upon arrival, Nurse Luciano placed the woman on a stretcher. I was shadowing him during triage.

Signora Emma was wrapped in a white sheet with her bare legs poking out, revealing intricate webs of swollen veins. Both rails of the stretcher were pulled up to prevent her from falling out. Signora Emma was contracting her left arm and lower lip in an unnatural way. The left side of her body appeared to be sliding downward. The ambulance crew who delivered her to Nurse Luciano reported that she had probably fallen out of her bed at the nursing home where she lived. The nursing home staff claimed they did not know how it happened, a not improbable case of negligence given the severe understaffing that nursing homes often endure. Signora Emma might have suffered a concussion, but the doctor who worked at the nursing home was not sure. Doctors who work in nursing homes are often very young—nursing homes tend to be doctors' first temporary assignments. In the view of many health care providers at the hospital, this meant that they were too inexperienced to be trusted.

Nurse Luciano called signora Emma's name, touching her gently on the shoulder. She remained silent, totally absorbed in what looked like pain, but this could also have been the distraction of dementia. Her eyes were not reddish, which meant that no evident sign of concussion was detectable. Was she just an unresponsive elderly woman with dementia?

"Wonderful!" said Nurse Luciano sarcastically to me after we had moved away from signora Emma. "If we don't know how she looked before the fall, how can we know what has changed?" The nursing home staff did not know exactly; they did not have any prior CAT scans to use as a reference for comparison. The ambulance crew reported on signora Emma's past history of neurological issues (she had had a stroke a year previously) and on her use of benzodiazepines to treat depression. Signora Emma had neurological difficulties of all sorts: she could not speak properly, her mouth was twisted, and her left arm was held in an unnatural position. But none of this could be trusted to pin down an emerging acute state of either stroke or concussion. All the signs Nurse Luciano observed might have resulted from the previous year's stroke.

Since there clearly was no way of knowing what signora Emma looked like before her presumed fall, Nurse Luciano decided to wait for her relatives to arrive, in the hope that they might provide a clue. In the meantime, he assigned a yellow code (a high-priority code) to her, so as not to take any chances. She needed a priority CAT scan.

What Nurse Luciano really feared was that signora Emma had been sent to the hospital to die. It was far from unknown for elderly care institutions to attempt to avoid medicolegal troubles by sending critically ill or aging people to the ER as emergency cases, even though they were suffering from chronic conditions that could not be treated there. This was another reason why Nurse Luciano and his colleagues in the ER tended to mistrust reports coming from nursing homes. The fall could have been a mere excuse to admit a dying old lady.

After two hours, signora Emma's family appeared at the reception. It had been a month since they had last seen her, so they were unsure as to whether she looked any different. Nurse Luciano concluded that they could not be trusted to help him decide whether the old woman had had a stroke or a concussion.

Soon after he spoke to signora Emma's relatives, the CAT scan results were returned, revealing no concussion. At that point, Dr. Roberto, a young but experienced practitioner, had to decide whether to admit signora Emma to the hospital or discharge her back to her nursing home. It was not possible to improve her medical situation. On the other hand, in his conversations with signora Emma's relatives, Dr. Roberto later told me that he had gotten the impression that her relatives did not trust him and were rallying a protest in the event that he refused to admit her to the hospital. Dr. Roberto decided to dodge the problem by hunting for a bed for the elderly woman to die in under the care of nursing staff in the solitude of a hospital ward.

WHEN HEALTH CARE PROVIDERS MISTRUST PATIENTS

People who visited the ER regularly developed important health expertise. Arianna, an eighteen-year-old woman with a thick crown of curly scarlet hair and a lean face framed by wide, round glasses, is an example. For three months, Arianna had experienced unusual pain that started in her left leg and went up her back, all the way to her head. This pain produced intense migraines. Suffering from a condition that no medical professional seemed able to identify, Arianna and her mother, signora Margherita, tried to juggle between various explanations.

Arianna told me, "I always get new symptoms. And despite having undergone so many medical examinations, no explanation has emerged." She glanced at her mother, who sat next to the stretcher where Arianna had been placed in the inner corridor of the ER.

"Often doctors tell me, 'Go to this other specialist, or to this other.' Sometimes I feel like a *palla rimbalzata* [bouncing ball] tossed between different medical services," she said, frowning. "No specialist can tell us anything precise. We looked on the Internet. Me and Mum do a lot of research on the Internet. This is why we now believe it could be mercury related."

Arianna's mother interrupted her. "Some doctors say it's fibromyalgia," she explained. "But she's only eighteen, and she hasn't had any trauma or anything, so . . . People on the online forum say try dental decontamination from mercury-based dentistry materials. Some dentists treat cavities with mixtures containing mercury, you know. That could trigger chemical effects that seem to be like her symptoms. Also, she had three cavities treated at the same time her symptoms started. So now I'm looking for a *dentista biologico* [a dentist who only uses products that contain no chemicals, like ceramics] to do a dental decontamination.[10]

"So we'll try that too," the mother continued. "I don't believe it is fibromyalgia." She sighed. "It's so unfair. . . . she is very young and should not be continually suffering like this."

Arianna did not think that she had many options to find help for her pain, apart from coming to the ER when she was suffering in order to receive a vial of painkillers infused directly into her vein. But she was vexed by how doctors treated her. Because her suffering did not fit any diagnostic category, she was often asked to undergo psychological treatment or psychiatric evaluations. She had submitted to both multiple times, with no results. Psychiatrists ruled out any pathological traits. The psychologist made her participate in group therapy that Arianna told me she enjoyed, but her suffering did not improve.

Arianna could anticipate most of the doctors' questions. With impressive precision, having learned a great deal from her experience of receiving so many different diagnoses, she told doctors exactly what they needed to know. She was a regular at the ER, coming often to relieve her symptoms and get further tests. Whenever she came to the ER, she always brought with her a thick ring binder full of official records, with a long index of examination results.

What Arianna did not guess on the day I interviewed her, as she was lying on the stretcher, was that Dr. Roberto, the same physician who had examined signora Emma, decided to tacitly infuse a placebo into her vein. Dr. Roberto wanted to test whether Arianna actually was suffering or if, instead, she perhaps just wanted recognition for something else.

After a while, Arianna told the doctor that she felt her pain receding thanks to what she believed to be the infusion of painkillers. To Dr. Roberto, Arianna's reaction was proof that her disturbance was of a "functional" (that is, a psychological or social) nature. What Arianna needed, the doctor decided, was to be put in contact, once again, with mental health professionals to address her suffering.

Dr. Roberto's decision to assess Arianna's suffering by using a placebo was not intended to disrespect her suffering. On the contrary, Dr. Roberto told me that he was trying to ascertain what Arianna "actually" needed. Furthermore, if Arianna had felt her pain growing more intense as a result of the placebo, the doctor would have swiftly infused a real painkiller. But even if carried out with the best intentions, Dr. Roberto's method of assessing his patient relied on a tactic of deception.

Deception here is indisputably a mode of power. In her research on lying in doctor-patient relationships in France, the anthropologist Sylvie Fainzang noted that "where power is given to the doctor and denied to the patient, the lying of the first expresses his way of exercising it, whereas the lying of the second expresses his way of taking it" (Dongen and Fainzang 2005, 48; Fainzang 2015). The power exercised by Dr. Roberto allowed him to assess his patient's needs, even as it accommodated her request for a painkiller. Deception as an expression of mistrust toward Arianna's suffering allowed Dr. Roberto to distance himself from Arianna's self-diagnosis so that he could decide how to treat it. Deception also had the effect of removing Arianna and her mother from the decision-making process. Neither of them was consulted in the doctor's decision to administer a placebo instead of a real painkiller.

On the one hand, Dr. Roberto's deception was a way to manage the unpredictability and complexity of Arianna's condition. On the other hand, to address Arianna's medical condition Dr. Roberto scheduled her for other external specialist appointments. So Dr. Roberto's doubt about (i.e., his mistrust of) Arianna's expression of suffering resulted in him entrusting someone else to address her situation (or passing her on to someone else, depending on one's perspective). Dr. Roberto was thus able to undergo a hidden triage that avoided open conflict with Arianna and her mother.

WHEN MISTRUST IS MUTUAL

ER staff who were skeptical of people's expressions of pain were also aware of the necessity to play along with them. As the anthropologist Els Van Dongen (Dongen and Fainzang 2005) described in her research in a mental health facility in Holland, many staff members were aware that patients' dramatizations or explicit deceptions may express "complex social and psychological struggles." In such cases, deception was a strategy to "survive unbearable and disgraceful situations" or a way of "resistance against" social exclusion (Dongen 2003; Dongen and Fainzang 2005, 109).

The case of signora Diana, a woman in her early seventies, illustrates this point. During an unusually warm and sunny morning of mid-November, signora Diana was escorted by two ambulance volunteers to the inner waiting area. Dressed in a threadbare pink dress and looking around searchingly with blue eyes nestled in a mat of wrinkles, signora Diana slowly limped her way up to the glass barrier, holding her lower back with her left hand. She explained to me and

Nurse Patrizia—who I was shadowing that day—that she had fallen over on a bus the previous day.

"Someone pressed the stop button too late, and the driver had to brake so fast that I fell on my butt. I couldn't hold onto the rails. I'm too weak," she said. She went home and took some paracetamol, but, she said, "Even if I took a thousand pills, *non conta* [it wouldn't make any difference] at all. The only thing *che conta* [that works, that makes a difference] is Contramal [a powerful opioid]. But my idiot GP took those away from me. What should I do? Should I be suffering all my life?" Signora Diana explained further that she had gotten *abituata a* (used to) Contramal because she suffered from vertebral fractures and spinal cord compression.

"I just want to stop suffering," she repeated. "You know, I am also diabetic!"

Nurse Patrizia nodded and assessed signora Diana as a green code. Upon receiving her code and a brochure that explained what it signified, signora Diana kept standing near the glass barrier, anxiously peering at us inside.

"I could have given her a white code," Nurse Patrizia whispered to me. "She is always here asking for painkillers!"

What did we really know about signora Diana? Triage interactions ranged from between three to fifteen minutes and were almost completely focused on evaluating a short-term temporal scenario (the emergent, the "here," and the "now"). The structure of interactions in the ER did not facilitate health care providers' possibilities of understanding patients' reasoning and their experience of suffering. The capacity of the ER to meet people's needs, to understand what *conta*—that is, what matters—was subordinate to its capacity to make sense of people's state of immediate vulnerability.

A clinical line of reasoning and an approximate timeline can be drawn from the triage interview in order to portray signora Diana's state of vulnerability. The encounter produced six factors that Nurse Patrizia deemed relevant to an evaluation of signora Diana's health needs.

First, the vertebral fractures and spinal cord compression underscored signora Diana's history of suffering and her past use of painkillers.

Second, diabetes was another clinical risk factor. It indicated signora Diana's dependency on care and a long history of involvement with health services.

Third, signora Diana's dismissive comments about her GP suggested that she found it difficult to access what she considered to be appropriate care.

Fourth, her reported fall on the bus indicated that she was an elderly woman who had difficulties balancing. This in itself clinically excluded the allocation of a white code. A trauma reported immediately after the fact was considered to be at least a green code since there was a major risk of it worsening within the first forty-eight hours. Signora Diana's case therefore required being given at least a green code, without any contact fees.

Fifth, having taken paracetamol suggested that signora Diana was a responsible person who did not just run to the ER at the slightest pretext.

And finally, sixth, signora Diana's limp and her nervous lingering around the glass barrier indicated that she felt anxiety and was suffering.

All these factors helped shape a linear narrative of events that decided the urgency evaluation. Clinically, Nurse Patrizia did not consider it feasible to give signora Diana some light palliatives. As signora Diana was already used to powerful painkillers such as Contramal, the drugs available to the triage nurse for infusion (ketoprofen or paracetamol) were of no use: ketoprofen or paracetamol would have been "like giving her *acqua fresca* [fresh cold water]," ER staff used to say. The only way to soothe signora Diana's pain was for her to see the doctor quite soon since the strong opioids she apparently was used to were allowed only under medical prescription.

Because the ER was not very busy on the day signora Diana came, she ended up waiting only half an hour before the nurse invited her to come to the other side of the glass barrier. When she entered the office of Dr. Carmen, the expert emergency physician on shift that afternoon, signora Diana sketched a different narrative from what she thus far had revealed. She started repeating her story about falling while on the bus, but then she suddenly turned to her real concern: the Contramal. When Dr. Carmen asked for further information, she explained that her psychiatrist, whom she had not mentioned previously, had advised her GP to cut off her strong painkillers because signora Diana was possibly genetically predisposed to dementia. The psychiatrist had informed her GP that opioids could trigger the development of dementia. To this, signora Diana added that she had fibromyalgia and an abdominal hernia that her GP had not taken care of.

"So, while I am here, can I also ask you for an X-ray for my hernia?" she wondered.

Dr. Carmen replied, "You know, we cannot use the ER for routine checkups. Let's start with an X-ray of your lower back, which is where you got hurt, then we will see."

At that point, signora Diana left the office and went to the inner aisle to wait for the X-ray. Dr. Carmen turned to me. "She is here because she is addicted to opioids," she said with a sigh. "Her GP lied to her about the genetic predisposition to scare her off with the painkillers' side effects. She probably takes them a lot."

I asked Dr. Carmen if she was going to prescribe any painkillers for her.

"Yes, because of the fall," Dr.Carmen said, giving me a knowing look. "I will not leave her without them. But I will change the type of opioid, so that her GP will not complain."

While she was waiting for her X-ray, I interviewed signora Diana in a secluded corner of the inner corridor. She explained to me what Contramal meant to her. She told me about her difficult childhood, where back pain was a constant concern, then of the major depression she suffered after the death of her first son, a few months after he was born. After her first episodes of anxiety and depression, she started drinking and taking Valium. Right after that, she was diagnosed with fibromyalgia and started taking Contramal. In that period, her father died too. Then, she had vertebral fractures and spinal cord compression.

"Now, I am 144 centimeters tall. Before the compression, I was 158! I was so beautiful back then. I was only forty [years old]!"

The only thing that could control her suffering was Contramal, signora Diana insisted. She admitted to having had dizziness and other side effects, but in the end, she said, "It is my life and I should decide. It is the only thing that works for me [che conta]. Should I have to suffer my whole life? Is that right?" Signora Diana continued: "I come here because I trust them [the ER]. I trust them. So every time I have a problem, I come here to solve it."

Signora Diana disregarded the possibility that the ER existed only to deal with medical urgencies. She trusted the ER to address her routine health issues. By personalizing her care regime, she understood the ER as taking the caregiving place of her GP, whom she mistrusted. But even as she professed trust for the ER, signora Diana nonetheless clearly felt it necessary to omit some parts of her story to better fit the urgency criteria of the ER and to use the doctors at the ER to bypass her GP and obtain a new prescription for the Contramal medication she so desired.

In signora Diana's story, trust and mistrust are in a mutually constitutive relationship. Disbelieving her GP, signora Diana turned to the ER, where she misled the nurse who conducted triage in order to be admitted. She seemed aware of the fact that her GP had a point in preventing her from overdosing on Contramal. As she herself admitted, she experienced dizziness and other side effects from the painkiller. But she still wanted it, and so, when coming to the ER, signora Diana omitted the reason why her GP had stopped her prescription for painkillers, instead insisting that she was there because of a fall on the bus. Having had extensive experience with the ER, signora Diana created a narrative in line with urgency allocation criteria by disclosing concordant signs and hiding discordant ones.

Mistrust structured both signora Diana's foregrounding of her fall, triage nurse Patrizia's initial suspicion, and Dr. Carmen's realization that signora Diana was indeed at the ER for the opioid Contramal. An important point here, though, is that this scenario of mutual mistrust did not hinder the establishment of a shared ground. In this case, it actually enabled it, crafting an alternative economy of attention amid triage negotiations.

By performing a clinically relevant vulnerability, signora Diana described her situation without directly asking for a new prescription of Contramal, which, if expressed explicitly at that point, would likely have been denied. This strategy set the scene for a silent understanding between signora Diana and Dr. Carmen concerning the doctor's responsibility to somehow address her patient's chronic suffering. Dr. Carmen immediately recognized this necessity, even though she was skeptical of signora Diana's narrative about the fall. Given signora Diana's desire to tailor her care, Dr. Carmen also engaged in a double agenda: addressing signora Diana's narrative as though she believed it while actually pursuing the secondary aim of mediating between signora Diana's longing for Contramal and Dr. Carmen's medical diagnosis.

Did signora Diana really fall on the bus? Who knows? The time line she recounted during triage evaluation vanished as soon as she was granted entrance to the doctor's office. She turned the ER into a place for routine checkups and requests. She affirmed her own idea of well-being, without openly challenging the health care providers' reference frame. Through a game of the said and not said, ambivalence on both sides facilitated a meta-communication, an economy of attention, to flow between two very different ways of understanding vulnerability. This does not mean that a shared agreement about what was urgent was reached. In fact, the opposite was true. Within a space of duplicity, two competing understandings of what was urgent were able to coexist without being reduced by one another or developing into a full-fledged conflict (as we saw happen in chapter 4 between Dr. Paolo and signora Gianna). In signora Diana's case, the relationship between a layperson's needs and expert knowledge was at once iterated and subverted. Dr. Carmen's capacity to decide over urgency remained intact, and signora Diana obtained her painkiller.

WHEN PATIENTS MISTRUST HEALTH CARE PROVIDERS

Mistrust offered the possibility of assessing and potentially finding new economies of attention that impacted on triage. A close connection existed between the practices of "education" that we addressed in chapter 5 and Dr. Roberto's mistrust of Arianna's expression of suffering. Both aim at managing individual's requests for care that do not match clinical urgency in the ER, but in contrast to what we saw in chapter 5, where Nurse Monica chastised signora Tania about her inappropriate use of ER resources, Dr. Roberto was able to avoid an open confrontation with Arianna and her mother. In a similar way, Dr. Carmen and signora Diana's silent understanding can be taken as an example of improvisation, a makeshift solution to people's recurring (and in principle inappropriate) calls for help. Mistrust in this sense shaped an economy of attention that carried the potential to both control relations and silence them—as we saw in Dr. Roberto's move to disallow Arianna and her mother any say in his decision-making—but also to facilitate insight and creativity, as in signora Diana's case.

Over coffee at a bar near the hospital, I chatted with Lucia, a young triage nurse around thirty, about mistrust. We were enjoying the pale light of the late winter sun. Lucia's dazzling smile and wide clear eyes struck me as quite a contrast to my own pale, unshaven face and bloodshot, tired eyes, the result of the tight schedule of shifts I was following. Lucia worked similar shifts, but she seemed indomitable. Energetic as always, Lucia told me about her own experience seeking care, when everyone mistrusted her.

"I was sick, but no one took me seriously," she began. "Instead, they laughed and diagnosed me with *sindrome aviopriva* [literally, "bird deprivation," meaning "penis deprivation"]. It all started with a strong fever. I used to take a lot of paracetamol to deal with it during my work shifts. At one point I collapsed at work, so the ER staff decided to hospitalize me for four days for tests. It was the only four days when I had no fever at all." She shrugged her shoulders and smiled ruefully.

The "diagnosis" that Lucia mentions, *sindrome aviopriva* (or *aviopenica*) is a jocular label that both female and male health care workers apply to women who suffer from something that seems to have no medical basis. "Penis-deprivation syndrome" suggests that the real problem is that the female sufferer just needs to get laid. The mix of Latin (*aviopriva*) and medical jargon (*sindrome*) makes this dismissive joke sound like a genuine medical diagnosis.

Even though "penis-deprivation syndrome" was bandied about as a sexist witticism, a more serious subtext to the diagnosis is that women who came to the ER, more often than men, were thought to misrecognize or even invent their symptoms as a way for them to deal with a life that they found dissatisfying for other reasons. Misrecognition of women's suffering played out along more general patriarchal power structures of Italian society, where women have lower salaries, are entrusted with unpaid care work, hold less prominent positions and more precarious jobs, and often have to choose between career and family (Yanagisako 2002; Krause 2009).[11] There was no equivalent "diagnosis" for men. In this sense, the mistrust that the ER staff directed toward patients frequently had a gendered target.

Lucia continued, telling me that "some of the staff thought there was nothing wrong with me. I asked a nurse once if she would hand me a thermometer to take my temperature when I felt my fever rising, but she just snapped, "No, *we* [i.e., the hospital staff] will take your temperature"—as if they suspected I would falsify what I saw on the thermometer."

Lucia rolled her eyes. "Finally, they let me have an MRI [magnetic resonance imaging—a procedure in which radio waves and a powerful magnet are linked to a computer to shape detailed images of inner organs] to make me happy so that I'd be convinced that I really wasn't suffering from anything medical at all."

Actively mistrusting Nurse Lucia's self-diagnosis that something was wrong with her, the object of contention became her anxiety rather than a possible medical problem. Not exhibiting clear signs or symptoms, the inner hospital staff relied on a stereotype of a hysterical woman to explain her behavior. Her worries were dismissed by the clinical decision-making, described as anxious fantasies.

But Lucia did not give up. She refused to believe that her symptoms were just figments of her imagination. "I went to the radiology department to look at my MRI results," she told me, "and I self-diagnosed. I knew some concepts of oncology, and I saw what looked like a mass, a vascularization. I diagnosed myself from zero. As soon as I was released from the hospital, I went to look for help in other hospitals and private clinics." After almost a month, the department of radiology where Lucia had had her MRI scan called Lucia back and told her that, upon closer examination, there might indeed be something that might merit a closer look. Lucia told me she replied, "'You really do not understand, do you? Tomorrow, I am getting surgery for it!'

"They filed my medical records dismissing me as the *aviopenica* without actually looking at what I really had," Lucia said. "Their mistake was huge. I wanted to talk with the head of that department, but I was too focused on saving my life at that time. I felt alone. And I learned from that experience never to underestimate a patient's complaints. It happens at times during triage, when you evaluate someone *tutta gnè gnè* . . . all wah, wah, wah, with perfect makeup, a chic haircut, and a fashion-model attitude. All the talk: 'If she was really in pain she wouldn't be wearing makeup' and the like. I received it myself. It was hard to get listened to.

"I remember one doctor once upbraided me, telling me that it seemed like I *wanted* to have cancer. 'Here, *we* decide who has cancer and who doesn't,' he said. 'And you have nothing!'" Lucia continued, telling me that she felt cast out, alienated, when she experienced her colleagues' mistrust and with so many doors being slammed in her face. She began to understand why people tried to skip the line in the ER to get care and be listened to. Every time she went to a new specialist, Lucia presented herself as knowing she had cancer. When the diagnosis finally arrived, she felt liberated. The doctor told her that yes, indeed, she had a rare form of malignant cancer. She told me that she exploded in a sigh of relief, to his complete surprise.

"The most difficult thing," she concluded, "was to be diagnosed and listened to."

Finishing our coffee, I asked Lucia, who, remember, was a triage nurse who worked in the ER, how cancer had changed her way of approaching patients. She told me that on a professional level, it always made her particularly supportive of those kinds of patients. Once, she told me, a young woman came in with a port (a small silicone appliance inserted beneath the skin to facilitate blood samples and injections). A colleague of hers did not know how to handle the port, so he asked Nurse Lucia for help. She knew everything about it, partly because she is a nurse but also because, when she had had cancer, she had had one herself. This woman had cancer as well, and she was in a state of complete despair. Sensing this, Nurse Lucia told the young woman that she had cancer too.

"I told her that I was still receiving treatment, and she looked at me with big surprised eyes. I looked fine and was working at the hospital, and I could see that impressed her. She asked me how that was possible. I told her, 'Look, things could have been better, but here we are. We walk and breathe. You have a boyfriend who loves you no matter what. You have a group of relatives and friends all waiting for you outside.'"

That young woman, Lucia told me, stepped out of the doctor's office with a completely different attitude. Before, she was "goggle-eyed like a goatfish" (due occhi da triglia). Now, hope sparkled and made her shine. The doctor who examined her was about to prescribe antidepressants, but when she came back and saw the young woman, she changed her mind. She looked at Lucia and asked, "What have you done to her?" Lucia gave me a knowing smile. "'I just disinfected her port,' I said."

Feeling close to seriously ill patients, Nurse Lucia understood many of their concerns. In a sense, she found herself in a halfway position between the caregiver and the patient. In this example, the young woman with cancer received from Lucia what other caregivers had been unable to provide: hope for control over her upcoming future with cancer. Nurse Lucia's experience of mistrust toward the health care staff who overlooked her case allowed her to intuit and trust the stories of seriously ill patients. Lucia's experience of being distrusted triggered her capacity to question. Doubt turned into agency, practical and embodied, allowing Lucia to imagine what could have been different and how, for both herself and for the seriously ill patients she later attended to as an ER professional.

But this did not come without a price.

Nurse Lucia told me that she now worried that she concentrated too much on seriously ill patients, whom she could understand better, at the expense of other less serious cases. She admitted to mistrusting many of those. Even though Lucia was herself distrusted, she could not avoid mistrusting people whose suffering she thought was exaggerated in relation to her own experience as both a patient and a nurse.

What this shift of attention underscores, as experienced by Nurse Lucia, is first that a mutually constitutive relation existed between trust and mistrust in the ER, something we also saw in signora Diana's interaction with Dr. Carmen. But most importantly, Nurse Lucia's account also shows how mistrust created an economy of attention that still had to deal with the fact that attention was a limited resource in the ER. In practice, this could create a new space for care, but as Nurse Lucia' s newfound biases implied, a new arrangement of attention also produced new areas of neglect. Nurse Lucia told me herself she now disregarded some of the calls for help from patients she believed had less serious troubles than the ones she had experienced herself.

MISTRUST AND CARE: A NEW ECONOMY OF ATTENTION IN THE ER

Mistrust in the ER is not an inherently bad thing. It is, rather, a tactic with practical effects amid care arrangements and outcomes, some arguably negative, others arguably affirmative. For instance, Dr. Roberto was able to diagnose Arianna by withholding information and deceiving her, ultimately perhaps directing her to more effective care than a vial of painkillers would have provided. Signora Diana's mistrust of her GP drove her to the ER, where she ultimately succeeded in obtaining the opioids she desired to manage her pain. Dr. Carmen's mistrust of signora Diana's narrative established a compromise between her own diagnosis and signora Diana's felt needs.

The exercise of mistrust also compelled patients to contest health care providers' decision-making and resist their diagnoses. Nurse Lucia's refusal to trust her medical colleagues' diagnosis of her condition drove her to seek out alternatives—in this case, private health services. Signora Diana is another example of the same dynamic, using her mistrust of one segment of the medical establishment (her GP) to seek alternative services in another (the ER). Mistrust and trust in practical care situations stand in a mutually constitutive relationship.

In respect to how urgency was supposed to be negotiated, according to the ER staff, mistrust created new ways of directing attention between patients and staff. It facilitated diverse modes of making a difference in the ER. Anthropologists have long described how the practice of medicine creates and governs difference. By detailing global inequalities of international medical knowledge production, examining disparities in the response to wide-scale disasters, or addressing the daily organization of patients' clinical charts, they showed how triage draws the line between care and indifference, the visible and the invisible.

Mistrust in the ER made a difference in subtle ways that could at once make visible or mute people's calls for help that the ER staff felt in principle did not belong there. Triage is increasingly evolving around conflict between staff attempts to maintain medical authority and patients' efforts to seek care. The exercise of mistrust became a way for experienced patients to create space to maneuver without openly challenging the ER's clinical urgency criteria. And for the staff, mistrust allowed them to enforce triage, even as they deftly avoided open confrontations with patients. Mistrust facilitated a workplace ethic that avoided conflict.

But as the experience of Nurse Lucia showed, such avoidance did not prevent the formation of areas of neglect. The case of elderly signora Emma, who arrived at the ER from her nursing home, is an example of neglect, in the sense that the ER practitioners (like, possibly, the nursing home staff) were so focused on avoiding lawsuits that they were never completely honest with the old woman's relatives about what actually could or could not be done to help her.

This ethic of duplicity, doubt, and silent understandings fit a triage that found itself at an impasse. Both the reinforcing of medical authority (in the case of Dr. Roberto and Arianna) and improvisation and creativity (as with signora Diana and Dr. Carmen) could unfold without ever reaching a shared agreement about urgency. Within spaces of ambivalence, opposing perspectives on urgency could coexist without developing into full-fledged conflicts.

But even though mutually constitutive relations between mistrust and trust created ways to avoid conflict in the ER, they did not extinguish them completely. Violence was a daily presence in the ER.

7 · VIOLENCE AND ITS CONSEQUENCES

Alcune persone sono come bombe a orologeria. Non sai mai quando esplodono.

(Some people are just like ticking time bombs. You never know when they are going to explode.)

—Interview with a triage nurse

Everyone I asked among the ER staff agreed that violence in the ER was on the rise. They all blamed this surge on the impasse that I have been documenting: on the predicament that arises in the ER when people present for assistance with problems it is not designed to handle and where health care providers are therefore confronted with precarity that they simply cannot resolve.

In the ER, violence was both verbal and physical. The ER staff told me numerous stories about times they were shouted at, threatened, kicked, or hit by drunk, disturbed, or noncompliant patients. The violence could also be more serious, as when an outraged patient threw a fire extinguisher at a nurse or tried to stab a nurse with a knife after being forced by the police to come to the ER.[1] Once, I witnessed a visibly drunk man, who did not want a blood sample taken, punch a young nurse in the face. Another time, a male nurse was kicked violently in the stomach by a woman high on drugs, who shouted at him to go f-ck himself (*Vaffanculo!*) when he carried her out of the ambulance. I was present when a belligerent professional boxer knocked out three members of the ER staff before being sedated with an injection of valium. Family members, too, can be violent, and there have been reports from several regions in the country of health care providers brutally assaulted by outraged family members when they were informed of a patient's passing.[2] And according to the Italian nursing union, NURSID, "4% of nurses have been held at gunpoint at least once during their career."[3]

Like the rise in patients who seek out the ER for problems that are not assessed as clinical urgencies, violence against ER health care providers is not just an Italian phenomenon. In the United Kingdom, figures issued by the Health Services

Advisory Committee reveal that 50 percent of all cases of violence against professionals occur in the ER (Saines 1999). In the United States, research involving 3,465 ER nurses revealed that 25 percent of them had been subjected to more than twenty acts of aggression during the previous three years (Gacki-Smith et al. 2010).[4] Triggers of violence vary from excessive waiting times, waiting room conditions (e.g., extreme noise, cold, or heat), alcohol and drug abuse, hostile attitudes of the ER staff, patient anxiety, lack of information, and the absence of alternatives to ER care (Hodge and Marshall 2007).

ER violence is regularly underreported by health care practitioners, who tend to minimize trivial episodes. Yet violence against ER staff regularly makes the headlines in Italian newspapers. One study of nurses conducted in fifteen hospitals in fourteen different regions of the country, out of the twenty regions in total, suggests a dramatic national picture: 90 percent of the ER nurses interviewed had been subjected to verbal violence, 52 percent had witnessed an assault on colleagues, 35 percent were victims of physical violence, and 6 percent had suffered serious injuries that took more than fifteen days to heal (Ramacciati et al. 2019).

Violence against ER staff, perhaps predictably, has been fodder for far-right politicians. In 2009, the Lega Nord political party attempted to link such violence to the supposedly unruly presence of migrants in the ER.[5] The party campaigned to force hospitals to report people with illegal migration status and to institute a police presence in the ER. More recently, in August 2020 the (center-left) government passed a law that increased criminal penalties for perpetrators of violence in the ER (which ignores what actually gets people to the ER) and created a national unit for monitoring violence against health care workers (decree n. 2117/2020).

During fieldwork, episodes of violence occurred mostly in the triage assessment area because this was where patients were crowded together, waiting for medical attention. Families and friends of red-code patients were allowed to remain in the waiting room near the triage area, and they sat there anxiously awaiting news. Because the ER lacked an alternative space, a patient's passing or other distressing news was often communicated there. Even more than its actual occurrence, the potential that violence might erupt made health care workers pay attention to particular gestures and attitudes of patients. Potential violence constituted an event that had to be anticipated and, ideally, prevented by the ER staff (Adams et al. 2009). This resulted in a not insignificant amount of attention and time being devoted to people identified as potentially violent—attention and time that needed to be managed in relation to the already limited amount of time that health care providers were able to devote to triage practice. In this sense, violence and the potential for violence were important factors that influenced how urgency was negotiated in the ER.

PAYING ATTENTION TO VIOLENCE

It was a Tuesday morning of a dazzling spring day. Patrizia, the triage nurse I was shadowing that day, was absorbed in her task of evaluating patients, complaining about the multitasking required by the job, as she prepared a copy of a patient's document. The waiting room was unusually quiet, but the atmosphere was brittle. Everyone seemed convinced that peace was not going to last. When I commented on the ER's unusual serenity, Nurse Patrizia looked up from her computer and quipped, "Wait until the lunch break. Around twelve it's gonna get messy."

As if fulfilling this prediction, two members of the ambulance staff and two Carabinieri officers (the Italian military police) suddenly appeared through the ER entrance near the internal waiting cubicles, escorting a tall bald man around fifty. He looked exhausted. His face was hollow, and he walked lethargically. He was dressed in a bathrobe, which opened to reveal scruffy boxer shorts and a stained undershirt.

His eyes, though, were fiery, wild and red and angry. He clenched his fists tightly, displaying swollen veins on muscular forearms. His wide shoulders arched slightly upward, making him look like a boxer entering the ring. Nurse Patrizia regarded him through the glass door and instructed the ambulance staff to place him in a wheelchair in front of the glass barrier.

By that time, I had been in the ER long enough to know what placing someone in front of the glass barrier meant: he was dangerous.

Stories about violence were widely shared among the staff and helped create a common narrative about which people were regarded as dangerous and hence who was accorded particular attention and placement in strategic spots of the ER, such as in front of the glass barrier. The main perpetrators of unpredictable violent reactions were widely assumed to be (1) drug addicts (particularly users of drugs such as cocaine, methamphetamines, and heroin), (2) mental health patients, (3) openly belligerent people, (4) elderly people suffering from Alzheimer's or other dementias, or (5) alcohol-intoxicated loners. In addition, there was always danger when people arrived at the ER in the aftermath of violence, such as physical fights, car accidents, any sort of harassment, suicide attempts, or crimes such as murder.

Attention given to potential violence in the ER had a strongly gendered dimension. In the stories the ER staff told, perpetrators were mostly male. The assailants or potential assailants were often sturdy and scary, either semiconscious from drugs or alcohol intoxication, or aggressive and nasty, swearing and yelling. On the other hand, to be the victim of violence often carried a component of femininity. Female members of the staff were thought to be at greater risk of being victims of violence than men, even though I personally witnessed more than one male nurse and male doctor being punched or kicked by female patients. And when male nurses or doctors were subjected to assault, they not infrequently asserted their masculinity by saying something like, "If that had happened outside the ER, I would have really let them have it."

Of course, violence in the ER was not only an "invading" force that had an impact on the staff. In many senses, violence was also part of the everyday life of the ER (Das 2008, 294–295), and it was tied to institutional care practices in multiple ways. Biomedical and psychiatric care practices can be experienced by patients as violent (Garcia 2010; Mulla 2014; Stevenson 2014). Care practices can have violent side effects, including repression, misrecognition, and harm. They can involve exclusion, biases and racialization, or discrimination on the basis of ethnicity, class, gender, and sexual orientation.[6] Or violence can be deliberately used to protect the health care staff and their practice when strategic to, and closely linked with, law enforcement or military action (Varma 2020; Cook and Trundle 2020).

But the immediate enactment of violence was felt mostly by the ER staff, and the hospital had instituted some measures to protect them. Hospital security guards, for example, were available and could enter wards at the request of staff. A security guard once told me that the most important part of his job was to keep up appearances: to have a certain *cipiglio* (frown). The preferred pose was chin up, looking down at people from head to toe. He and other security guards struck this pose as they performed a firm military walk in full shiny uniform within the ER waiting room. Or they stood still like ancient Roman statues, hands on their waists just above their belts, ostentatiously close to the black leather cases that held their pistols.[7]

The ER staff had an ambivalent relationship with these security guards, and with law enforcement officers more generally, because they were sometimes thought to hinder the accomplishment of good care with their threatening presence, particularly where undocumented migrants were concerned. But at other times, the staff required their intervention—for example, when people started to act aggressively.

The ER staff were no strangers to the use of force. Sometimes people with dementia or who were under the effect of alcohol or drugs were forcibly restrained in order to draw blood or to prevent them from falling off stretchers. Screams, punching, and running were not uncommon reactions by people who resisted. Heroin addicts who wanted to enjoy their high, or alcoholics happy with their buzz, often rebelled against the injection of substances intended to counter the effect of drugs and ethanol.

"I've paid for this stuff!" they scolded the ER staff.

But no shouting or evident signs of violence came from the man who, at Nurse Patrizia's instructions, had been placed in a wheelchair in front of the glass barrier. He put his head in his hands and started to sob.

SHIFTING TRIAGE

"Ora è vostro" (Now he is yours), one of the two Carabinieri police told Nurse Patrizia and me in an official tone, after we joined them in front of the glass barrier. "He had a bad family fight, and it's not the first time." We learned from the ambulance staff that the man was named Massimo and that he had tried to kill himself by wrapping his bathrobe belt around his neck after a long violent fight with his elderly mother.

Nurse Patrizia measured signor Massimo's vital signs. She did not ask for more details about the situation. She was more interested in the immediacy of his clinical urgency and of assigning him a color code. His heart was racing fast. But that was normal after an altercation and an attempted suicide. Signor Massimo's acrid sweat also suggested liver problems.

As the last ambulance staff member walked away, he placed a hand on signor Massimo's shoulder, whispering "Coraggio" (be strong, literally, "courage"). Then signor Massimo was left alone to cry. He was placed in what was known in ward jargon as *il parcheggio* (the parking lot): one of the six inner cubicles where people awaited a doctor's examination.

Nurse Patrizia went back to the reception and phoned a psychiatrist. She was following procedure for cases of attempted suicide: psychiatrists had to be alerted right after triage. They were required to leave the psychiatric ward where they worked and come down to the ER to conduct an assessment. Nurse Patrizia was particularly anxious to fast-track signor Massimo. She immediately classified his case as a yellow code and even decided to prioritize him over other patients who had been given the same color code. Urgency was given to signor Massimo not primarily because of his clinical condition but because of his assumed *ingestibilità*, the impossibility of managing him during waiting and his potentiality to become violent. Nurse Patrizia also checked his clinical records in the hospital database: hepatitis C, a past of major depression, ex-alcoholic and heroin addict, off drugs for ten years. Having just attempted suicide, being an alcoholic and former heroin user, suffering from mental distress—all this immediately classified signor Massimo as a potential *bomba*, a bomb on the verge of a violent explosion.

The person-bomb metaphor was widespread in the ER to convey high unpredictability of a person's behavior. But attention to "ticking bombs" (*bombe a orologeria*) also revealed an important subtext: triage was a vulnerable process, and it had to be defended. To do so, health care providers' attention was directed away from clinical urgency and deflected to protecting themselves and their possibility of carrying out their clinical work. In this sense, violence reconfigured the economy of attention that paced ER staff activities.

Such situational improvisation of triage differs from the changes that the anthropologist Harris Solomon (2017, 2022) described in the casualty ward where he worked in Mumbai. Solomon details the situational changes to which triage was exposed in relation to unstable resources such as a severely restricted number of ambulances or a lack of stretchers or blood reserves (2017, 350–351). In the Italian ER I am describing, changes in triage were not so much tied to available clinical resources as they were oriented toward the anticipation of potential violence, which could interrupt or derail clinical practice. A change in how attention was distributed, from the evaluation of clinical urgency to the focus on potential violence, is what Nurse Patrizia enacted when she evaluated signor Massimo.

People categorized as ticking bombs required particular techniques of paying attention. These techniques of attention were geared toward deterring potentially violent patients from harming themselves and others and preventing them from hindering triage activities. The techniques were not part of ER staff formal training, but they were widely shared. One such technique was to isolate the bomb-person in strategic spots of the inner waiting area, where staff were able to watch them, as Nurse Patrizia did with signor Massimo.

Other techniques involved distraction. Potential bomb-people were offered a coffee or a cigarette to smoke outside the hospital facility. Occasionally, troublesome patients were invited to have a brief chat so that a nurse could discover what staff defined as their *chiave*—their relational key—the way to connect with them and make them feel attended to. Chats about hobbies served this function, as did questions about vacations or favorite music. Much as a professional explosive defuser would tinker with a prospective bomb, staff in the ER tinkered with people to switch off potential violence.

REVEALING ABANDONMENT

But was signor Massimo really on the verge of exploding?

Soon after Nurse Patrizia phoned the psychiatrist, I escorted signor Massimo into the doctor's office in the yellow-code area. The two Carabinieri followed me, but after a quick gesture by Dr. Alberto, the ER physician on call that day in the yellow-code area, they remained outside the office door.

Normally, ER physicians on call waited for the psychiatrist to come down to the ER before allowing a waiting patient to enter their office. But even though the psychiatrist had not yet arrived, because of Nurse Patrizia's insistence, signor Massimo was directly fast-tracked into Dr. Alberto's office. This was another technique that staff used in their dealings with individuals they considered as potentially violent. Besides granting urgency, this arrangement also facilitated a longer time for examination, precious time that could allow a better understanding of a potentially problematic patient's situation.

As I closed the office door behind me, Dr. Alberto invited signor Massimo to sit on the stretcher. He asked signor Massimo what had happened, informing him that the psychiatrist was on his way to the ER to speak with him. "I don't need a new psychiatrist; I already have mine. I am not the problem here," signor Massimo said, looking directly at Dr. Alberto. The doctor nodded in response as signor Massimo finished his sentence: "As long as my mother's ghosts keep haunting her life, I cannot live any longer."

In a stream, signor Massimo's words flowed swiftly, telling his mother's story. She was the daughter of a woman who had been constantly beaten and raped and who was forced to marry her rapist after she fell pregnant to repair her family's shame (an Italian practice known as *nozze riparatrici*, "repair marriage"; see Herzfeld 1980), toward the end of the Second World War. Massimo's mother ferociously hated all men, especially her father and her only son, in whom she saw her own rapist father.

Signor Massimo told us he had spent his life trying to gain his mother's respect. This respect, he said, was withheld even now, when he alone was taking care of her because her mobility and independence had increasingly declined with age. All this he did while he worked as a bartender with a short-term employment contract. Signor Massimo's mother preferred his sister, who, he said, did not care about her and frequently asked for money, which his mother gladly gave her.

Mother and son argued continually about his sister's behavior. That morning, the morning of the altercation, in a dispute about his sister, signor Massimo's mother had challenged him, shouting "Cupem! Cupem!," meaning "Kill me! Kill me!" in the local dialect, implying that since signor Massimo would never succeed in changing his mother's mind about his sister, he might as well murder her. Signor Massimo almost took his mother up on her dare. He beat her badly, leaving her lying on the floor of his apartment. Horrified at what he had done, he called an ambulance and locked himself in the bathroom. He took five doses of his antidepressant medication and attempted to take his life with his bathrobe belt. "Did you hang yourself?" interrupted the nurse on duty in the doctor's office. Suicide attempts were often a source of know-how curiosity in the ER. "There is no need; there are other ways . . ." Signor Massimo left the phrase suspended while everybody's eyes moved from his face to the almost engraved neat purple mark that necklaced his throat.

While signor Massimo was telling this story, another nurse was engaged in a seemingly futile quest to find a vein in his arm to draw blood. Situations like this often arose with elderly patients or with current or former drug addicts. Before the nurse could call the anesthesiologist—the only kind of physician thought of as being better than nurses at finding "good veins"—signor Massimo calmly took up the task himself, locating a vein and inserting the needle on the first attempt.

Massimo's mother—who had been sent by ambulance to the other hospital in the city—was expected to recover from her injuries, and she decided not to press charges against her son.[8] Social services were alerted. Apparently, social services were already well acquainted with this dysfunctional situation. Signor

Massimo waited in the ER until the afternoon to speak with another psychiatrist, who simply referred him back to his own therapist so as not to further fragment his already troubled relations with care institutions.

Rather than an explosion of violence, what signor Massimo revealed was a long history of violence that dated back to World War II. It involved tangled brutal events through three generations and raised the problem of how to break a chain of violent normality (Das 2006, 9–16; Mulla 2014). In this case, violence was framed not by the exception of a potential explosion, as Nurse Patrizia initially feared and as violence was often interpreted in the ER. Instead, signor Massimo's detailed explanation of his and his mother's situation was a rare case in which scattered pieces of people's lives became articulated in a comprehensive narrative that became intelligible to the ER staff.

Exposing a different temporality and causal chain of events upon which the assault on his mother and his attempted suicide needed to be understood, signor Massimo was able to convince health care providers that he did not need another psychiatrist or further medication that targeted his psychological state. His needs could not be addressed by a biomedical approach. Instead, they were symptoms of a violent normality of social abandonment (Biehl and Eskerod 2005; Das 2006).

The relevant relations went far beyond diagnostic labels and ER-specific ideas of who was thought to be dangerous. Signor Massimo's relationship with his mother, as he described it, superseded the category of perpetrator and victim. It assumed the shape of an ambivalent kinship relation of hate, violence, and dependency (see Mulla 2014, 176–194). The grounds for engaging signor Massimo's case in the ER became reframed from a focus on him as a threat to the ER staff to his compelling narrative, which addressed why the tools available to the staff were of little help to engage a family context of suffering that seemed to encompass almost a hundred years of violence.

IMPROVISING AN ALTERNATIVE TRIAGE

Signor Massimo's case exemplifies a plot twist. From being regarded as potentially dangerous, when he was listened to his needs became understood in a differently meaningful frame. The creation of such a space of understanding between people felt to be potentially violent and the ER staff had to be handled with particular attention. This attention often involved reshaping triage in an attempt to find a meaningful connection while keeping the potentially violent patients calm. Experienced professionals talked about the importance of finding people's relational *chiave*, their "key," in order to understand their suffering more fully and to productively negotiate urgency.

Professionals were not equally skillful at such attempts, and many had specific preferences about the types of patients they felt able to connect with. For instance, thirty-four-year-old triage nurse Flavia had extensive experience with humanitarian aid projects, in addition to a passionate love for the African continent, to which she traveled whenever she had the opportunity. She always immediately volunteered to deal with so-called difficult patients of African descent. Another triage nurse, Lidia, told me that handling unpredictable patients means the following:

> You need to be humble. You have to recognize when your presence or what you can do is not helpful, and then you have to call someone else that could instead find that person's *chiave*. For instance, I have never experienced any trouble with male patients, but once I could not find a connection with a woman who was angry with all the good-looking ladies, including myself. It is like when you are dealing with patients with autism. It's never you who chooses the autistic patient; it's the autistic patient who chooses you. And if that patient doesn't trust you, you must step aside. But if she trusts you, you alone get the *chiave* through which people open up, and you become the one that has to care for that person. It doesn't matter if you were assigned to another ER area, you need to switch and adapt rapidly, or that patient will tear the doctor's office to pieces in your absence. People come to trust you if you show them you are not afraid. Even if someone glares at you with bloodshot eyes, you have to face them directly. You have to go past the glass wall and know exactly when the moment will be that they lash out. Only right before then do you run for cover. The more you try to bridge gaps and work around fear, the better chances you have of finding people's *chiave* and becoming therapeutic.
>
> For instance, I remember once there was a South American woman who beat up two male cops. The police locked her in the doctor's office where I was working. She threw anything she could find at me; she desperately wanted to hurt me. I didn't have much information about her apart from the fact that she was visibly drunk and outraged. The cops just told me that she had had some love trouble with a man. So I looked straight at her and made it clear whose side I was on: "You are right to be angry. Men are all assh-les!" And that was our click. I started talking shit about men, and she visibly calmed down. Then, the cops came back into the office, and she tried to punch them again, so we had to hold her down and inject her with a sedative. The morning after, when she had recovered from her massive intoxication, she was crying desperately because of what she had done. She had attempted suicide by running onto a freeway.

As many members of the ER staff, particularly triage nurses, described it, finding a person's *chiave* meant negotiating urgency in a particular way. It implied a certain degree of reflexivity, first about the caregiver's subjectivity (i.e., gender, ethnicity, and life experience) and the possibility of engaging meaningfully with others' understanding of what was therapeutic (as Nurse Lidia described) and, second, about the patient's subjectivity and biography. Finding a person's *chiave* involved assessing needs not against a biomedical standardized body—like triage was supposed to do in the ER—but by letting them emerge in the course of interaction. Practically speaking, this meant that care in the ER shifted from being "anonymous"—that is, based on risks connected to a standardized body—to being focused upon people's different living conditions (Stevenson 2014, 7). Finding a person's *chiave* foregrounded the diversity of people's exposure to harm and the unequal embodiment of violence in their lives (Farmer 2004; Lock 2017, 5).

As important as seeking such connections was, though, the extensive attention granted to individuals like signor Massimo or the angry Latin American woman described in Nurse Lidia's story could not possibly be granted to everyone who came to the ER. Attention was a limited good. This meant that many of the patients who came regularly to the ER had to endure long waits and received little response to their needs since they were often regarded as irrelevant to the ER's definition of urgency. Some of these patients erupted into violence.

An example was the long hours that mental health patients had to wait after panic attacks, psychotic crises, or even suicide attempts because their situation was deemed less urgent than physical issues that could indicate a potentially rapidly worsening situation. Local mental health patients' and families' associations I spoke with highlighted the implicit undervaluing of the urgency of mental distress during ER triage procedures because "mental" and "functional" emergencies were less accessible than emergencies of a physical nature.

Other recurrent problems were experienced by people with cognitive impairments or decline. That was the case for signora Rosa, an elderly woman of eighty-six, who lay wrapped up in white sheets with her bare feet pressing against the pulled-up bed rails in the waiting area beyond the glass barrier. Signora Rosa looked at me intently with bright-green eyes. I smiled at her and at the blonde woman sitting beside her, who turned out to be signora Olga, her daughter, who had brought her mother to the ER from the nursing home where she lived.

Several hours had passed since she had arrived with her mother, signora Olga told me, and they were still waiting to be examined by a doctor. Her mother was growing increasingly impatient. She was not used to being handled by strangers, and she was visibly restless. She resisted attempts to insert an intravenous drip into her arm. She pulled out the needle twice and threw the bandages used to secure the drip on the floor.

Signora Rosa clearly just wanted to go home. It simply did not matter how many times her daughter explained to her that she had fainted that day at the nursing home and so she needed to be checked in the ER; signora Rosa wanted to go home.

Signora Olga told me that her mother wanted to follow her usual routine at the nursing home: moving around with her walker, listening to music with her friends, and singing. As suggested by the anthropologist Jong-min Jeong, even though physicians frequently regard repetitive routines like these as abnormal pathological behavior, such routines carry an affective capacity for people suffering from dementia. Through repetition, they are able to control their world, maintaining their subjectivity by iterating gestures and interactions with others in a reassuring, careful manner (Jeong 2020, 4–8).

A triage based on the principle that people are all vulnerable in the same way and that difference is imposed by clinical risk could not make sense of the impossibility for a patient like signora Rosa to wait long hours like everyone else, of her embodied necessity to repeat gestures and not be prodded by strangers. Difference in this case manifested in the embodied way that signora Rosa lived with dementia and her routines at her nursing home.

But in contrast to what happened with signor Massimo, time and attention to finding a *chiave* could not be granted to signora Rosa. That day was particularly crowded, and elderly patients considered potentially violent by the staff were in general more likely to be left by practitioners to the care of their family members or, alternatively, left to wait on stretchers with bed rails pulled up to prevent them from falling off or going around the ER, hurting themselves or others. So, trapped on a stretcher with pulled-up bed rails, waiting for something she did not understand while strangers physically restrained her to prick her arm with a needle to take blood tests, she kicked, punched, and shouted desperately.

Patients with Alzheimer's or other forms of dementia often started screaming and struggling against pulled-up bed rails, risking injury to themselves by falling off the stretchers they lay on. Once they were finally admitted to the ER doctor's office, the usually long wait had already jeopardized any possibility of creating a meaningful relationship with ER staff—who were also untrained to deal with patients who required particular kinds of attention.

As we have seen, ER staff improvised alternative triage arrangements that gave more attention to people's biographies and conditions of living to find out how urgency could be negotiated on such a basis. Though these attempts were successful in some cases, as in signor Massimo's, this process required an extensive amount of attention that neither nurses nor doctors could normally provide to patients. Improvisation in the ER was provisional and fragile.

FRAGILE NEGOTIATIONS

One factor that ensured that violent or potentially violent people with mental health distress (like signor Massimo), intoxicated by drugs or alcohol (like the Latin American woman described by nurse Lidia), or affected by cognitive decline (like signora Rosa) were in the ER was because they had nowhere else to go. A considerable percentage of individuals thought to be potentially violent were what in wry ward jargon were dubbed *utenti frequenti*—that is, "frequent fliers"—people who went to the ER anywhere between four to sixty or more times per year (Grover and Close 2009; Doupe et al. 2012).

Some of these frequent fliers eventually formed a connection of sorts with staff members. The ER became the place where the attention that had been withdrawn from them by state biopolitics could partially be reinvigorated. But such a possibility was always the result of delicate negotiations. To achieve this connection, some particularly cunning people tried to get themselves classified as bomb-person characters to be attended to during crowded ER moments. This strategy seemed most available to people who had experience in dealing with the ER and who had figured out that becoming difficult was a way for them to directly influence the attention they could receive.

At the beginning of a Tuesday night shift in April 2018, one such savvy bomb-person appeared in the ER. The waiting room that evening was busy, and the two triage nurses on duty were trying to stay focused, even though the waiting list was getting out of hand. Doctors were slow in conducting their examinations that night, which resulted in nurses having to deal with escalating malcontent. Twenty-eight people were waiting, and the nurses' replies to their insistent queries about when it might be their turn became more strident as new patients arrived and the number of people in the waiting area kept growing.

At this point, signor Franklin was escorted into the ER by the volunteer ambulance crew of the emergency service. Signor Franklin, a thirty-five-year-old homeless man from Ghana, was a frequent flier well-known to Nurse Antonia, the triage nurse I was shadowing that evening. The ambulance volunteers escorted him to the glass barrier. Sitting in a wheelchair, signor Franklin swayed unsteadily. He had an absent look and was wearing dirty clothes and worn-out shoes.

The ambulance volunteers waited while Nurse Antonia finished evaluating a gasping elderly woman in the third cubicle of the inner waiting area.

"They found him in the street running around aimlessly, so someone called us," one of the ambulance volunteers told her, referring to signor Franklin. "He looks drunk but doesn't smell of alcohol. Do you know him?"

"Yes, I do," Nurse Antonia answered. "You can go," she said, dismissing the volunteers.

As soon as they turned and left, she asked signor Franklin: "Hey, Franklin, do you want to talk to somebody?" He nodded distractedly and then looked away.

Nurse Antonia knew from past experience that signor Franklin was not easy to deal with, first, because he fell into the category of people thought of as potentially violent but mostly because he usually required a lot of attention—attention that Nurse Antonia could not afford right then. As she later told me, her main concern was to make sure that signor Franklin did not interfere with the other triage tasks she had to fulfill, particularly as it was an exceptionally busy evening. Thus, she wanted to call the psychiatrist in to take care of signor Franklin so that she could dismiss him from the triage area.

She left signor Franklin in his wheelchair in front of the glass barrier and the triage reception desk, in the same strategic spot where Nurse Patrizia had put signor Massimo to wait. There, signor Franklin could wait for the psychiatrist under her supervision while she prioritized other tasks.

But just as Nurse Antonia was about to return inside the glass barrier, signor Franklin fell out of the wheelchair, heavily, and lay on the ground blocking the entrance to the ER. Nurse Antonia and I ran out to see what had happened. As soon as we arrived, signor Franklin started screaming and crying desperately. I started speaking English to him, asking "What happened? Where does it hurt?" He cried, "Everything hurts! Please, doctor, kill me!" "I'm not a doctor," I told him. "I'm a researcher, but I can translate what you have to say to the nurse so that she can help you!" "Can you ask her to kill me? Please!" he screamed.

Refusing to stand up, he fought off everyone who tried to help him. Nurse Antonia went to help another incoming patient and left me kneeling beside signor Franklin, trying to talk to him. Two ambulance stretchers were now waiting outside the ER, trying to get in behind him. After a little while, he got up onto his knees in the middle of the room and shouted out loud: "Kill me! Please, can someone kill me? My father has died! Please, kill me!"

At that point, Nurse Antonia stopped the injection she was about to give to an elderly man lying on the stretcher in cubicle four. She came up to me and whispered, "He always does this. He is not drunk. I know what he is looking for." She went back to the inner corridor and returned to signor Franklin's side with a stretcher. She asked him gently if he wanted to rest. Signor Franklin wiped his tears with his right hand and got up. Helped by us, he lay down on the stretcher. Soon after, we heard him snoring quietly.

Stunned, I asked Nurse Antonia what had just happened. She explained:

Three years ago, his father died in Africa, and he has never recovered. Sometimes Home Help [a local association that helps refugees find accommodation] throws him out onto the street because he is a hothead, they say. When he doesn't know where to go, he comes here. Since there is so much going on here right now, I cannot deal with him any other way. So, I will let him sleep.

The drama enacted by signor Franklin seemed intended to make him visible, creating an urgency in order to bypass the ER's usual economy of attention and provoke the kind of improvised engagement that we saw illustrated above with, for example, signor Massimo. Displaying suffering in a theatrical way and blocking a strategic passageway allowed signor Franklin to counter Nurse Antonia's attempt to apply the formal category of standard triage practice and classify his issue as psychiatric. She had already tried to accommodate signor Franklin's situation as an individual condition of distress that needed a mental health approach. Because she already knew his situation, she wanted to deal with it by having him speak to some-one about his personal issues.

But when signor Franklin fell in the crossroads of the triage area, screaming and refusing to cooperate, things started to change. There, the match between signor Franklin's situation and psychiatric care fell apart. Triage attention had to shift from a clinical definition of urgency to one that had to focus on signor Franklin's individual demands. He did not want to talk with anyone. He wanted a safe place to rest quietly. Having encountered him in the ER many times previously, Nurse Antonia knew that his *chiave*, his key, was his need to rest.

Because signor Franklin was a frequent visitor to the ER, I met him many times. He always seemed to look for a place to stay by himself, a place where he could sleep or mourn his father's death quietly and safely. This kind of safety and privacy could only be achieved by co-opting the ER's internal space and using a stretcher to lie down on. So he regularly enacted his drama to make his suffering visible and so to disrupt standard triage practice. This move produced a new urgency. Signor Franklin earned priority, and his desire to rest quietly on a stretcher was acknowledged and fulfilled. In this way, signor Franklin used his (in the eyes of the ER staff) "inappropriate" vulnerability productively. It could not be ignored, and it forced the hand of the ER.

Some health care practitioners labeled behavior like signor Franklin's as unethical and disrespectful of others' needs. But regardless of how they felt about it, signor Franklin's enactment of vulnerability opened a space for other kinds of requests to be heard. These requests pertained to fundamental rights that were largely left unattended by state authorities, such as access to housing, psychological help, and socioeconomic support.

Negotiations like the one that occurred between Nurse Antonia and signor Franklin prompted a practice of urgency that was more ample and more gener-ous than patients usually received. By co-opting the physical space of the ward, signor Franklin affected the ER's capacity to imagine urgency in relation to the daily forms of suffering and abandonment that faced many of those people who regularly returned to the ER. Of course, signor Franklin's behavior also created problems; by forcing attention to be focused on him, he temporarily wrenched control of the attention economy from the ER staff. Even though the situation was quickly recovered by Nurse Antonia, it illuminated a risk that undergirded staff anxiety about violence and violent people: What would happen if everyone did that?

The structural dilemma posed by people thought of as potentially violent, like signor Franklin, compelled a compromise between the ER's duty to address clinically urgent cases and its having become the last safe haven for an increasing number of people who did not have anywhere else to address long-standing suf-fering. People living on the street, like signor Franklin, could obtain in the ER a warm meal from the hospital canteen; rest on a stretcher from the fatigue of life in the street; take a warm shower within the rescue service headquarters nearby; or even obtain new clothes from a collection donated to the hospital by one of the local Catholic charities. All of this was increasingly dependent on nurses' and doctors' capacity and willingness to provide their limited attention.

The ER was not designed to cope with chronic ill health and compromised living conditions. But while it could not improve people's social and economic conditions, the absence of alternatives was enough to encourage people to return multiple times to the ER. But lacking systematic attention to his abandonment, what signor Franklin achieved that Tuesday in the ER was only a temporary exception to his existence framed by the shadow of violence. This structural violence ultimately could not be managed by improvised techniques of paying attention (Farmer 2004).

After completing my fieldwork in the ER, I kept in touch with Nurse Antonia and many other members of the ER staff. I continued collaborating with the staff to create a training course to discuss structural issues in access to care. It was during one of those moments of collective reflection about triage and urgency that Nurse Antonia told me some distressing news: signor Franklin had passed away a few months after I had left. He was run over by a car. Apparently, he was going back to the city center after having spent a night in the ER, walking in the gray morning light alongside a busy highway. No trains or buses were available that early in the morning, and he had no money for a cab. He used to get to the hospital by ambulance, and he would always walk back to the center, some fifteen kilometers away, on the exposed side of the road. The ER staff continually warned him against walking on the highway, especially at night.

But Franklin did not have any alternative.

CONCLUSIONS
The Negotiation of Urgency

> If there was a way to make people feel attended to [*ricevere attenzione*] when they enter the ER, to make them know that someone cares for them, then we would have solved all of our problems.
>
> —Head nurse of the ER

Anthropologists often write in the "ethnographic present" about the people with whom they work and the situations that unfold. One reason is to create a sense of immediacy; another is to attempt to bridge the distance in time between what was observed during fieldwork and what appears after the material has been analyzed and written up. Even so, the chronological distance between what was observed and what is finally recorded in an anthropological account means that all ethnographies are always already history.

The ethnography of the Italian ER that I present in this book, it turns out, became history unexpectedly quickly.

On 20 February 2020—slightly more than a year after I concluded my fieldwork—Annalisa Malara, a thirty-eight-year-old anesthesiologist working at a small hospital in Codogno, in the region of Lombardy, northern Italy, diagnosed a man of her own age who would become known as *paziente uno*, the first case of COVID-19 in the country.

"I thought of the impossible" (Ho pensato all'impossibile),[1] the anesthesiologist later told the media, recalling how she had to fight against hospital protocols to be allowed to send the man's nasal swab to a specialized laboratory in Milan for diagnostic examination.

The results came back—the man had tested positive for SARS-CoV-2.

Suddenly, COVID-19 turned from being a distant disease linked to the consumption of exotic creatures like pangolins sold as food in the wet markets of a faraway Chinese city to an alarming Italian (and soon afterward, global) reality. In Italy, the failure of contact-tracing procedures and the rapid spread of COVID-19 led to rushed political decisions culminating in a strict national lockdown, an attempt by Italian authorities to contain the first wave of what shortly after (on 11 March 2020) would be declared a pandemic by the World Health Organization (WHO).

The national lockdown in Italy originally lasted for eight weeks, from 9 March until 3 May 2020. The regions of Lombardy and Emilia-Romagna (where I conducted fieldwork) were two of the hardest hit nationally, registering a staggering total of more than 20,000 deaths within two months. Italy would reinstitute strict regional lockdowns multiple times in twelve out of the twenty regions of the country throughout 2020 and the following year, including in Emilia-Romagna, until vaccination rollouts became widespread toward the end of 2021.[2] In May 2023, when the WHO declared the end of the health emergency, Italy had registered over 187,000 deaths nationally directly associated with or caused by COVID-19. This is some 30,000 deaths more than civilian victims of World War II.

From the beginning of the pandemic as it spread in Italy, hospital overcrowding was "breaking news." The level of patient saturation of ERs and intensive care units and the lack of available beds were broadcast relentlessly, filling everyone with dread. Virologists, epidemiologists, and experts of all kinds routinely appeared in national media, voicing a wide array of often wildly divergent opinions about the virus' behavior and its impact on people's lives and on the health system.

Attention—who and what deserved it, whether the local and national economy or citizens' health—was at the forefront of discussion and concern, and this focus on attention highlighted both the country's precarious social and economic fabric and the intense vulnerability and inadequacy of the Italian health care system. The word "triage" started to pop up in mainstream media. It became a topic of vitriolic debate.

Considerations about triage such as those I have foregrounded in this work provide a perspective that allows us to interpret some of the social and political processes that were involved in the Italian response to the COVID-19 pandemic. As I have described it, triage is about the negotiation of urgency. Triage involves the circulation of attention, resulting in the shifting and always vulnerable making of difference. Triage—like the organization of health care, the spread of the virus, and the public health response—is therefore always inherently social, and understanding how it works as a process calls for social considerations. Focusing on economies of attention, such as the one that I have proposed, facilitates an analysis of the mutually constitutive relations that both enmesh and structure the ER, the hospital, and the broader social context of people's lives.

This focus contrasts actively with the tendency of biomedicine to approach an emergency like the SARS-CoV-2 spread as a nonsocial matter, in which context the health response should be solely based on a strict monitoring of individual behaviors (Raffaetà 2020; Quaranta and Bodini 2021). Such an approach allowed policy-makers to blame preventable deaths on the "inappropriate" behavior of individuals, rather than on the lack of coordinated national public health measures or other wider social and economic factors that increased the vulnerability of some to severe illness and death.

In this book, I have demonstrated that such an approach is inadequate, blinkered, and wrong. What happens in situations of emergency, as within the ER, can work as a prism to illuminate inequity within the broader Italian society and its changing welfare state. I deployed the analysis of health care governance and triage as a systematic example of how the analysis of attention helps us situate the effects of and the response to complex phenomena, like a pandemic, within local social dynamics. Core to the interactive reshaping of people's cognition and social reality, attention helps us make sense of micro and larger-scale political economic factors that result from structural inequalities, austerity measures, and, in this case, the pandemic.

My fieldwork was conducted prior to the outbreak of the pandemic, but the different chronicities, the impasses, and the conditions of precarity that I discuss became even more intense in this new situation of urgency.

As SARS-CoV-2 became the new urgency upon which all attention and resources were directed, patients like many of those I described in the preceding chapters, who had nowhere to go apart from the ER, were effectively cut off from care. The impasse of triage I have described did not vanish. Rather, the circuit of people returning to the ER resulted in even more serious outcomes. People who needed care for chronic conditions such as dialysis for kidney failure, chemotherapy for cancer, or routine checkups for cardiovascular diseases or diabetes were made to wait as medical resources were directed to COVID-19 cases. People, wary of infection and shocked by the rapid escalation of deaths in Italy, avoided seeking medical care. People who suffered from chronic conditions saw their health status plummet. The ER staff told me that many of their habitual patients had diabetes degenerating into necrosis of limbs. Unchecked heart conditions escalated into heart attacks. Chronic kidney stones developed into sometimes life-threatening blockages.

Needing care, people with noncommunicable long-term conditions all eventually resorted to going to the ER—they had nowhere else to go—and their seeking for attention turned into a rush for immediate lifesaving treatment. But within the hospital, overworked staff had to improvise with inadequate organizational arrangements, worsened by more than ten years of budget cuts and austerity measures (Alfieri et al. 2022).

Overcrowded, understaffed, and under intolerable pressure, hospitals became sites for the massive spread of contagion, as patients who suffered from noncommunicable conditions ended up becoming infected with COVID-19, spreading it, and, in many cases, dying (as predicted by Manderson and Wahlberg 2020). The fragility and inadequacy of the Italian public health care system was on public display, in all its harshness and inadequacy.

Such fragility, I argue, was compounded by the fact that many people had nowhere else to go apart for the ER. The ER remained the only public place always open where people knew they would, eventually if not immediately, gain attention.

Although this ethnography quickly became history, the analysis that emerges from it allows us to shed light not only on the pandemic, but on the new direction that health care is taking in Italy, as elsewhere. The ER provides a unique perspective on the political economics of health and illness and the management of need.

A CHANGING HEALTH CARE

The ER generally and the triage area particularly—with its border-like environment and its thick glass wall—is a crossroads between the hospital and the lives of ill people. As we have seen throughout this book, people who sought care were frequently aging, lonely, or excluded, their lives influenced by harsh social and economic conditions. The ER's attraction was informed by promises peddled by pharmaceutical companies and private medical practices. In the context of the increasing marketization of health care, the ER was a key space of conjunction between the state and the life of citizens. It was a space of conflict and bargaining, where different understandings of what deserved immediate attention mingled and clashed.

A variety of media reports portray the overcrowded ER as a place of acute crisis. But the ER, flooded with people with chronic conditions, rather illuminates the quotidian misery that arises from social and economic precarity. It was the place where people went to try to patch up a partial recovery after surgery, to skip long lines for specialists' consultations, and also, sometimes, to try and find shelter for the night in the midwinter cold.

Frequently co-opted by people for what health care providers dubbed "inappropriate use," the ER attracted individuals who encountered obstacles to care seeking and who found their needs unmet. Whether it was a troubled relationship with their GP, a lack of access to primary care, insufficient funds to pay for private alternatives, or despair over the long wait required to see a specialist or have a diagnostic test, needs like these streamed into the ER.

Health care providers' work routines structured around urgency were not well adapted to the tangled experiences of suffering with which nonurgent patients presented and for which they sought acknowledgment and assistance. In this sense, the course of interactions in the ER occurred in a kind of gap in health care providers' possibilities of understanding each patient's reasoning and experience of suffering. ER professionals did what they could with makeshift solutions, but ultimately they were unable to meet the needs of many of the people who came to them seeking their attention. Of course, that does not mean that the staff did not save lives every single day. It means that they were continually being called upon to do much more than that. And they could not.

This situation could be and often is interpreted as a failure of the Italian welfare and health care system, just like the overall response to the pandemic. We saw that the Servizio Sanitario Nazionale (Italian National Health Service [NHS]) was only founded in 1978 and that, in principle, it promotes health and universal care coverage as "a fundamental individual right in the collective interest, and guarantees health care free of charge to the destitute" (article XXXII of the Italian constitution, 1948).[3] But what we have seen throughout this book is how in practice this principle is seriously compromised.

The conditions under which ER providers experienced great difficulties in addressing and making sense of people's suffering are not random. Such development went hand in hand, starting in the early 1990s and increasing after the financial crisis of 2008, with ER overcrowding worldwide. Unsurprisingly, the phenomenon corresponds temporally with the ascension of neoliberal welfare reforms while also correlating with the demographic shift toward an aging population and the epidemiological prevalence of noncommunicable conditions.

The Italian health care system in particular was freighted with compromise between the protection and promotion of people's health and the market imperative of growth. Directly inspired from the first universal tax-funded system in Europe, the United Kingdom's NHS established on 5 July 1948, it took Italy thirty years of heated political debate between the long-running Christian Democratic Party, the Socialists, and the Communist Party to design a much more decentralized and fragmented system than the UK prototype.

The introduction in 1999 of laws like "intramoenia," meaning the possibility of doctors working as private workers within the very same public facility, or "extramoenia," meaning their ability to work simultaneously within the public system and in private health care (see chapter 5), created an important conflict of interest within the one public system. These laws created the conditions for which doctors hired within the public system were able to perform the very same tasks either within the public system or within the private one, in which context they were paid between six and seven times more. These laws had an important impact on the lengthening of public waiting lists for medical examinations.

Moreover, the central gatekeeping figure of the general practitioner (GP) remained outside the public service because GPs are employed only as private contractors. This arrangement ensured the influence of pharmaceutical companies, local pharmacies, and private health insurance over GPs and their key role as prescribers of drugs, medical treatments, and examinations.

But ER working conditions were also made worse with the process of neoliberalization of the Italian NHS from 1992. Since then, the redistribution of national funding from the regions to local health units and hospital administrations has been based on how many diagnoses are made (Diagnosis-Related

Group). The more diagnoses, the more money the hospital or local health unit receives from the region as a refund of costs of treatment (including diagnostics, medication, and inpatient stays) and investment for future activities (see chapter 4). The fewer hospital admittances and the shorter the hospital stays, the lower the administrative costs and the more likely that people like signor Umberto, who we met in chapter 5—a patient with complex chronic vulnerabilities who was discharged very soon after kidney surgery—would come back, thereby generating a new, profitable diagnosis.

This cycle exemplifies how health care importantly turned into an instrument for market profit. This circular movement focuses not on meeting people's needs, nor on their right to health, but rather—in a version of the very same logic that Dr. Paolo identified in signora Gianna's customer-like behavior in chapter 4—on producing diagnoses as commodities. From the perspective of a financial framework like this, the ER, which has to face people's needs directly, is essentially a burden. The ER's financial budget is not based on diagnoses. It is fixed on the basis of the previous year's expenditure, even though the costs of operating ERs increase with overcrowding. A financial sinkhole, the ER is focused on risk assessment and not on producing diagnoses. Unlike other wards that are lucrative diagnosis makers, the ER is not profitable.

ERs are also key streamlining structures through which people are admitted to the hospital; their suffering can produce lucrative diagnoses for other wards. As the gateway of the hospital, the ER needs to be kept functioning. Yet the more underfinanced an ER becomes, the greater the profit a hospital structure gets in return. Impossible to be made fully profitable and unable to be completely shut down, the ER stands still as a thick place for attention in which people can negotiate what needs urgent public engagement.

Just like their incoming patients, though, ER wards nationwide receive only residual attention from hospital administrations that have the explicit mandate to contain the costs of health care and obtain financing according to medical performance. This means that hiring nurses and doctors in the ER is mostly dealt with by intermediaries (Italian, *cooperative,* literally 'cooperatives') to limit costs and maintain professional staff in posts under precarious working contracts, usually lasting only a few months. The precarity of newly hired staff, in addition to understaffing, has an impact on the ability of ERs all over the country to undertake long-term planning and train new professionals. Under the conditions that have ravaged public health care since the late 1990s, the professional lives of nurses and doctors in the ER have become very short—two years on average, in contrast with the lifelong contracts offered and still held by professionals like Nurse Patrizia, who started their careers before the process of neoliberalization. These newer professional lives are marked by bitterness, even though many ER staff are also understandably proud to make a "difference" to those whose lives they save in the ER.

As I write in April 2024, few of the professionals I met in 2017–2018 are still working in the ER. The vast majority of them have left for jobs without exhausting night shifts, the constant fear of violent aggression, and the persistent sensation of not having done enough for patients. In 2022 alone, 600 physicians in Italy left the ER, while the number of patients grew by 20 percent more than 2021. To keep this pace, the national association of emergency medicine (Società Italiana Medicina d'Emergenza-Urgenza [SIMEU]) explains that Italian ERs are understaffed by a staggering amount of 49,000 medical doctors and 70,000 ER nurses.

Igniting competition and facilitating the hyperspecialization of medical knowledge, with emphasis on multiplying detailed, lucrative diagnoses, the administrative framework in which ERs operate hinders collaboration between diverse hospital services. At one point, for example, an ER doctor told me that he and his colleagues had tried to create a "silver code," which would fast-track elderly patients incapable of enduring long waits. The silver code was intended to refer these patients directly to the geriatric ward for examination there. The geriatric ward, however, was not willing to renounce its privilege as an inner hospital ward that did not have to deal directly with incoming patients. Like other inner hospital wards, the administrators there were aware that a direct link with the ER would have meant substantially changing the geriatric ward's working routine. In times of financial shortages and increasing requests for hospital accountability, they declared that this was not an option.

As far as I know, the head of the ER did not reply with indignation to such refusal. He simply acknowledged his marginal role in the hospital administrative hierarchy. He knew very well that to break the ER's isolation, he had to look for alliances outside the hospital. But general practice clinics and primary care facilities were also increasingly underfinanced, and that was not an option. In a calm, matter-of-fact tone, he explained to me that the ER, just like triage nurses, was stuck between a rock and hard place, between people's increasing need for care attention and state and private interests' efforts to marshal such requests into lucrative diagnoses.

Exemplifying the broader change happening within the Italian welfare state, hospital administration profits financially from the growing distance between people's increasingly precarious lives and the capacity of primary health care or social services to respond to their needs. The increasing gap between people's experience of suffering and the fragmented state response is an advantage for a financial system based on diagnosis, rather than the protection and promotion of people's health. Their experience of suffering is erased in favor of, in this case, a focus on diagnostic procedures and economic cost-effectiveness.

While the state's public health campaign blames the "inappropriate use" of the ER by individual patients, the administrative framework in which the ERs operate creates the perfect conditions for ER overcrowding to continue and expand.

Moreover, an administrative framework that exacerbates attention over diagnosis at the expense of the protection and promotion of people's health fosters privatization of public health care. COVID-19 powerfully revealed such a trend, as the pandemic marked an intensification of privatization of health care in Italy. According to the RBM Censis report on private health care insurance of 2020,[4] 90.8 percent of the ten million Italians who participated in the study were dissatisfied with the level of service they received in the public health system. Private insurance companies and private hospitals' advertisements and television commercials increasingly targeted Italians' sense of insecurity, while those companies and hospitals simultaneously profited from care fragmentation.[5] One-third of the participants in the RBM Censis report (50% more than in 2019) declared that they wanted to purchase or already had purchased private health care insurance. Thus, the privatization of health care benefited enormously as a direct result of the Italian state's response to the pandemic (Armocida et al. 2020).

The process of neoliberalization starting in the early 1990s, the financial crisis of 2008, and the COVID-19 pandemic can all be considered as tipping points in the straining of the relationship between the Italian state and its citizens. The sociologist Jurgen Habermas (1975, 21–31) describes how welfarist states are increasingly at risk of breaking the existing compromise between addressing people's needs and the neoliberal market imperative of growth. He maintains that, trapped in this constant role of mediation between people's needs and the market's interests, states may fail to be seen as a "legitimate" interlocutor, one that people would trust to address their needs (46).

What I have illustrated throughout this book is that the people I have met in the ER in Italy do not feel seen by the state. By searching for staff attention in the ER, people struggled to make their individual needs visible to the state. This situation could be interpreted as an example of what Habermas calls a "legitimation crisis" (1975, 46–66). But even though in crisis, the ethnographic material analyzed here importantly shows how legitimation was reshaped in the negotiation of urgency in the ER. Simultaneously permeable and enclosed, the ER in Italy became the quintessential space to acquire visibility vis-à-vis the state, to negotiate what deserves an urgent public engagement.

ATTENTION AS AN ANALYTIC FRAMEWORK

With ever-decreasing available alternatives, an increasing number of people in Italy seem to seek out the ER as a kind of refuge. The triage performed there could be influenced, or subverted, in ways that interfered with what Foucault identified as the biopolitical dilemma of "make live" or "let die" (2004, 241). The impasse I have described for triage in the ER ensured that it never fully developed into either "letting die" (the exclusion from care altogether) or an active "making live" (full access to care that translates into dependable support). Triage was a recursive cycle of negotiations consisting of repeated requests and inconclusive solutions.

Due to the impossibility both for the staff to provide long-term solutions or exclude people completely from care and for patients to achieve satisfactory support for their long-standing troubles, the ER increasingly became a thick space for attention, at once a place of public relevance and of biomedicine.

As a core public place, the ER is, first, where nobody is left behind. It provides direct access to a wide disposal of resources like specialists, drugs, and medical examinations. Such radical universality of access creates a unique proximity between patients and nurses and doctors as frontline workers of a key state service.

By focusing on attention, in this book I have foregrounded how people's efforts to be seen by the staff—and more generally by the Italian state—meshed with the daily struggles of ER workers to do their job. They have to manage multiple requests at once, carry out the work they are entrusted with, and ultimately see and be seen by patients but also by their colleagues and their superiors in the hospital. This was the case, for instance, for Dr. Paolo, who, after his conflict with signora Gianna about her daughter's urinary tract infection, struggled to be acknowledged by the hospital administration.

Through an analytic of the modes of paying attention in the ER, I have illustrated the shifting dynamics of what Alice Street called the "everyday struggle to mobilize techniques of visibility" (2014, 227–232). Expanding on Street's insight, I have focused here on the flux, trade-offs, and mutually constitutive relations that create an economy of attention in the ER in a country, like Italy, subject to a profound transformation of welfare due to economic austerity measures.

By foregrounding the circulation of attention, the ethnographic material analyzed here shows how the everyday struggle for visibility in the ER is vulnerable to swift changes, in which hierarchies of visibility can be (re)negotiated amid the situational process of giving and receiving attention in the ward. This economy of attention is thus a microphysics of power that highlights how visibility, roles, resources, and ultimately urgency are unsettled and reshuffled daily by internal and external influences in the ward.

Highlighting the changes in the configuration of medical processes like triage, I have illustrated how the ER is also where the power of medicalization, as the making sense of people's problems through medical knowledge, can be reappropriated by patients. I have articulated this argument by demonstrating how attention constitutes an active counterpart of "visibility," a concept that, beginning with Michel Foucault's argument of the "birth of the clinic," has had an impressive fortune in medical anthropology scholarship (1994). Whereas visibility implies passivity—of a body objectified by the medical gaze—attention is an active resource that can be both bound to medical exigencies and bent to contextual happenings and people's emerging needs. Attention can be pulled away from its original purpose, and it can develop into improvised practices of care delivery.

Attention, as an active and limited resource driven by interactions in context, rather than visibility, as a boundary between the visible and the invisible that is established only by a single actor, redefines the focus of governing action in medical care. Attention shifts the key locus of production of knowledge about the other (visibility) from unilateral decision-making to the interaction with the other, who, even though in a state of subalternity, is nonetheless able to modify the way in which power is exercised.

This paradigm shift, first, reveals the importance of *decision-making contexts*. The context from being a passive element, such as the anatomic theater in the clinic described by Foucault (1994), becomes a lively, unpredictable setting where different human and nonhuman actors shape the conditions through which knowledge is produced. In chapter 3, for example, I described how triage is constantly redefined by its operational context, with rapid changes of scenario and multiple factors demanding the attention of patients and caregivers. As demonstrated here in the case of the ER, technologies, bodies, and subjectivities take a leading role in determining what kind of attention is possible in a care setting, with its dynamics, balance of power, and possibilities for interaction.

Second, foregrounding the analysis of interactions means to single out the different *priorities* that exist in decision-making contexts—priorities that determine interactions' timing, rhythms, and conflicts. Priorities vary depending on interruptions, changes in the context of interaction, and the possibility of giving attention to actors' purposes. Interactions are thus determined by context from which, in turn, different priorities take shape. These priorities and their conflicts emerge strongly in the ER in chapter 4, where I analyzed how the circulation of attention gives rise to a particular ecosystem of time that is, however, threatened by the presence of conflicting market interests.

The third element of an analysis of power based on attention as a heuristic is *value*. Just as different priorities develop from the context of interaction, different values and legitimacy of action develop from the unequal distribution of attention. Privilege and advantage are created for some and disadvantage and invisibility for others. In a recursive economy, what has value attracts attention, and attention creates value and legitimacy when it is directed toward a given object. In return, a change in value shifts power relations in place within a given context. This dynamic is exemplified in chapter 5, where the value of the claims of people referred to as inappropriate users in ERs is diminished by a public health rhetoric that is increasingly based on individual responsibility.

The economy of attention, which centers the analysis of power on interactions, reveals how the governance of self and others can be altered by changes in context, by conflicts in the construction of priorities, and by the influence that these have on the construction of value and hierarchies (see Figure 2). It reveals how improvisation plays a key role in contextualizing practices of governance

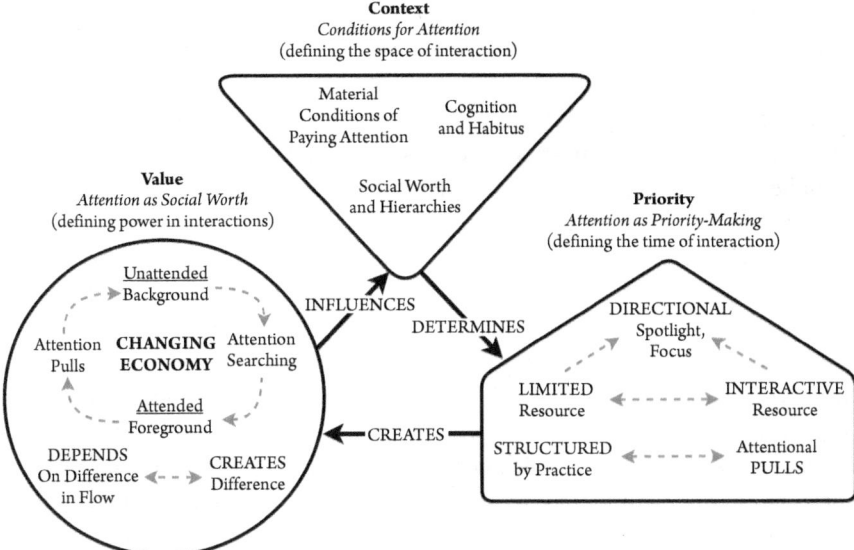

FIGURE 2. Schema summarizing the work of attention as a limited, interactive social resource

where attention as an active, relational, and limited resource plays a major role in constructing the right to care and its urgency.

UNEASY, CONFLICTUAL IMPROVISATION

An active paradigm based on the intersubjective uses of attention, rather than one based on a passive construction of visibility, advances anthropology's understanding of improvisation as the reshaping of medical governance in a precarious context. As this book has shown, the ER is a socially dense place where the effects of improvisation, of a different governance of care and attention, can be explored.

We have seen how friction occurred in the making of urgency. Clashes were difficult to resolve through compromise or "tinkering"—that is, a positive system of feedback in which the staff respond openly to the recipients' need for diverse care by working together to generate the best possible care with the means at their disposal (Mol, Moser, and Pols 2010, 10–14). As also noted by Catherine Trundle, tinkering care foregrounds positive aspects of improvisation by overshadowing challenges and limits within care (2020, 204). Limits in the ER were underscored by recurrent conflicts in daily negotiations of urgency.

As we saw, conflicts in making priorities in the ER frequently did not revolve around an accumulation of positive feedback. They developed instead from the recurrence of the unresolved tension between people's care seeking and staff attempts to maintain their medical authority. Uneasy and conflictual, improvisation in the ER prevented the triage system from collapsing even as it accommodated needs that otherwise risked being completely excluded from care. Both patients and providers were aware of the fact that improvisation was not only positive but came with a price. This included chronic waiting and unstable care solutions for patients and an impasse and increased stress, leading to work-related burnout, for ER staff, documented by an abundance of stress-related leave.

In her work on conflicts in care settings, Cristiana Giordano (2014) suggests that "translation" is better than "tinkering" as a way of apprehending how practical care affects bodies and subjectivity. Analyzing mental health interventions with migrant women, carried out by the ethnopsychiatry Centro Fanon in the northern Italian city of Turin, Giordano notes that "translation" implies a power asymmetry between translator and translated (2014, 10). The first has the power to reshape meaning, whereas the latter unavoidably must sacrifice some of its original essence, as an effect of the violence implied in any act of translation. Giordano illustrates that people's needs have to be made to fit into certain categories in order to be understood and attended to by caregivers and, more generally, to be reworked into the Italian state's discourse (2014, 10–11). She describes two logics of translation.

The first is "recognition"—that is, adapting others' understanding of what is to be addressed to preestablished categories of intervention, in a way domesticating and reducing the otherness of people's requests to one's own categories (Giordano 2014, 7). This first approach can be understood in relation to how psychologist William James describes the selective mechanism of attention, a spotlight that outlines the world according to a preestablished order amid the visible and the invisible (1950, 402–458).

The second approach identified by Giordano is "acknowledgment," in which caregivers recognize that they do not know for certain how to address people's requests. In recognizing this, caregivers adopt a more exploratory attitude. They turn attention into attentiveness, a form of openness to others' experience and plights (Petrement 1977). They attempt to engage difference rather than reducing it to sameness (Giordano 2014, 9–18).

The material I have discussed in this book affirms that translation better accounts than tinkering for what happens in the ER. An example is the case of signor Massimo, who attempted to take his life with a bathrobe belt. The long history of animosity between him and his mother, drenched in violence, inundated the categories of risk rating in the ER and confounded the ER's way of making sense of his suffering. Incommensurability in encounters with ER risk-rating categories was often experienced by mental health patients and by people like elderly signora Rosa and her daughter signora Olga, who were dealing with aging and Alzheimer's disease. The impossibility of making sense of long-lasting suffering through the categories offered by the ER, through what Giordano calls "recognition," was a source of friction and conflict between professionals and patients. But such conflicts at times triggered a more explorative approach in fitting the narrative of urgency in the ER, an "acknowledgment" of others' difference and an urgency unrelated to biomedical classification.

In a different way from that which Giordano describes, though, people with unmet needs who overwhelmed the ER were not only passive recipients of attention eliciting either recognition or acknowledgment. Although a power imbalance did exist, needs were negotiated and mediated in triage interactions, fueling conflict, certainly, but also driving attention away from preestablished categories of clinical urgency. By challenging the ER's priority-making and making its contingency visible, patients compelled new possibilities to get the medical staff to engage with their needs. Signora Diana, who crafted her illness narrative to fit a clinical urgency evaluation in order to obtain her longed-for painkiller, or signor Franklin, who heaved himself into the middle of the inner aisle of the ER, are two examples of how patients actively drew attention to and created new spaces for their needs to be addressed.

Even though mediated by biomedical ideas of the body and individual personhood, what happens in the ER is that triage—often represented as the pinnacle of medical authority—is turned into something more than a medical way of sorting. Medical categories in the ER are stretched, negotiated in context through the giving of attention to many more aspects of people lives that, in practice, get back to the ER to be addressed multiple times. Drawing legitimacy from biomedicine, people in the ER are able to reshape what deserves urgent public engagement.

Residual and yet increasingly central to many people's ever-diminishing opportunities to obtain health care and welfare, the ER has become a space of improvisation. We have seen how Dr. Elena carved time out of her tight schedule to coerce signor Stefano's sister into bringing him back home; how Nurse Lucia used her personal experience to convince a recently diagnosed young woman that despite her diagnosis of cancer, her life was not over; how Nurse Antonia settled signor Franklin down to sleep on a stretcher to grant him the privacy he was looking for. And so on. Needs that exceeded strictly biomedical interventions found a response in the makeshift, improvised space of the ER. There, agency, subjectivities, and care roles are negotiated in new original ways.

Insights from the lived experiences of both incoming patients and health care providers in the ER illuminate the ongoing changes within Italian welfare, as in many other Western liberal democracies. Such experiences show the ways in which the ER has turned into a thick space for attention as both a refuge and streamlining structure.

In the ER, biomedical tools and sense-making are confronted daily with their limits. But those limits are not only constraining. They are also enabling: they reveal people's creative capacity to use their suffering as a means of negotiating the economy of attention that shapes urgency within and beyond the ER.

ACKNOWLEDGMENTS

Nobody writes a book alone, and this monograph is no exception. It is a tremendous pleasure to be able to acknowledge the many individuals who have so generously enabled my efforts to describe everyday life in an Italian ER.

I dedicate this book and send my most heartfelt gratitude to the staff and the patients of the hospital where I spent a year of my life working and learning. In order to preserve their anonymity, I cannot list them by name, but with them I shared much more than an ethnographic project. I am grateful to everyone who offered me glimpses into their lives, either by talking with me in the ER waiting room or by allowing me to shadow them during entire exhausting work shifts, sharing with me hopes, concerns, and juicy hospital gossip. I am grateful to those who repeated their stories to me when I did not get it all the first time; who shared morning croissants and espressos after a long night shift; who patiently explained to me how clinical protocols work. I thank those dedicated staff members who spoke with me, with care and concern, after unsettling events, and for all the forbearing patients who ended my interviews with them with a sincere hug. I cannot thank you all enough.

I would also like to express my gratitude to the hospital administration and the Formazione, Ricerca e Innovazione office for having granted me access to hospital venues and for reviewing and evaluating my project. I am especially grateful to the hospital directory board, to the head and vice-head of the ER, and to the chief nurse. Your assistance, trust, friendship, and firm belief in my project enabled it from the start.

The fieldwork and the writing up of this book started up during my years as a PhD student at Uppsala University. I am particularly indebted to my main supervisor, Don Kulick, for all the ways he guided me to complete this project. This work owes so much to Don's insightful suggestions and keen eye for detail. Don engaged me in conversations that inspired and helped me develop many of the key analytical and theoretical concepts of this work. With his inspiring advice and countless corrections of drafts, Don has shown me what it means to be a good scholar and, not least, a good writer. His passion for anthropology, language, narrative, and descriptions will always inspire me.

My co-supervisor, Claudia Merli, provided many fascinating discussions about the most disparate theoretical arguments. Claudia opened up to me diverse analytical angles in my work for which I am much indebted. I am grateful to Claudia for always striking a balance between constructive criticism and supportive advice.

I wish to thank all the academic and nonacademic staff at the Department of Cultural Anthropology and Ethnology at Uppsala University for having made me feel welcome during my years as a graduate student and later as a postdoctoral researcher. Special thanks to Susann Baez Ullberg, who took the time to carefully comment on and engage with this book, and to fellow former PhD student Anna Baral for her enthusiastic support. I am, moreover, grateful to Mats Utas for his scholarly interest in my research.

The Engaging Vulnerability program at the Department of Cultural Anthropology and Ethnology at Uppsala University has provided me with exceptionally fertile ground to develop this book project. The stimulating interdisciplinary debates and innumerable seminars, courses, lectures, and events arranged by Engaging Vulnerability were key to developing this monograph. I am grateful for the many suggestions and the help I have received from Sverker Finnström, Maria Karlsson, Mahmoud Keshavarz, and Sharon Rider. They have inspired my work since I became a part of the program in 2016.

Mats Hyvönen deserves my special gratitude for all his help during these years in his capacity as a research coordinator of the Engaging Vulnerability program. Both an inspiring scholar and a very pragmatic person, Mats was always able to solve both intellectual and practical problems effortlessly.

My former fellow PhD students at Engaging Vulnerability deserve to be acknowledged for many inspiring conversations and both scholarly and practical advice: Vida Sundseth Brenna, Leyla Belle Drake, Carolien Hulshof, Macario Lacbawan, and Alexander Sallstedt. I wish to particularly express my gratitude to my fellow graduate students who joined the program at the same time as I did. My heartfelt thanks go to Adelaida Caballero, Karl Ekeman, Rikard Engblom, Erik Hallstensson, Kasper Kristensen, and Kristian Sandbekk Norsted for sharing your thoughts, your knowledge, your critical insights, your laughter, your beer, and your friendship: *Grazie mille.*

I also wish to express my gratitude to the participants in Don's writing seminar for commenting on some of the chapters in this book at various stages of the writing process: Clementina Amankwaah, Siddharth Chadha, Emy Lindberg, and Petra Östergren.

After my PhD, from 2022, this project was funded by the Swedish Research Council (Vetenskapsrådet) through my international postdoctoral fellowship. I am deeply indebted to members of the Center for Medical Humanities at the Department of History of Ideas at Uppsala University for welcoming me into their vibrant research environment. In particular, I would like to thank Ylva Söderfeldt, the director of the center, who commented on many of the book chapters and generously offered her wise counsel. Thanks to Ylva and Erika Sigvardsdotter, the center's coordinator, I was able to initiate several collaborative projects and broaden the lens of this book by conducting follow-up fieldwork on primary care during the third wave of COVID-19 in Italy.

I am thankful for my time as a visiting scholar in Bologna. I am especially grateful to Ivo Quaranta of the Center for International and Intercultural Health at the University of Bologna for encouraging me to pursue this book project at a very early stage. The final stages of writing benefited enormously from my time as a visiting researcher at the Interactive Mind Center at the University of Aarhus, where Mette Terp Høybye welcomed me and shared her incredible experience in applied critical medical anthropology.

As I transition to my current position as an assistant professor of social anthropology at the School of Global Studies at the University of Gothenburg, I would like to thank my new colleagues for their encouragement. I am particularly grateful to Maris Gillette, who offered her keen advice and impressive knowledge of Bourdieu's theory of practice to rethink my perspective on attention as a heuristic of power in social interactions.

Over the years, several scholars outside my home institutions have also provided me with valuable comments, counsel, and important input for this research.

Hannah Brown at Durham University generously offered incisive comments on an earlier version of this manuscript. Her feedback and thought-provoking suggestions have contributed greatly to the final form of this book. Ayo Wahlberg at the University of Copenhagen, with his insightful comments, inspired me to further elaborate my theoretical approach on attention. This work would also not have been possible without the generous scholarly interest and critical comments of Alice Street, at the University of Edinburgh, and the inspiration she provided for the development of the theoretical analysis. Her practical advice was also instrumental in my decision to approach Rutgers University Press.

I wish to thank Kimberly Guinta, former editorial director at Rutgers University Press; Nicole Solano, current editorial director; and Emma-Li Downer, publishing assistant, for their secure guidance throughout the editorial process. I am particularly indebted to Lenore Manderson, editor of the Medical Anthropology, Health, Inequality, and Social Justice series. From the early stages of turning my dissertation into a book to the final moments of writing this book, Lenore's keen eye for detail and unyielding trust in my project allowed me to continue to develop a sense of the book's trajectory and argument. Lenore's sharing of her immense knowledge of medical anthropology and writing was a real professional privilege.

I am obliged to the people who worked in the various parts of the production process that helped make this book possible at Rutgers University Press. I would like to thank the three anonymous reviewers whose generous criticism helped me develop the manuscript. Earlier versions of chapters 6 and 7 were published as articles in *Medical Anthropology* and *Global Public Health*, respectively. I would like to thank the anonymous reviewers for their comments, which helped to develop the text into the chapters of this book.

I would like to thank several members of the Medical Anthropology of Europe Network and Medical Anthropology Young Scholars for their helpful comments about my work. Thanks to Margret Jaeger for her input on our shared interest regarding the spread of violence directed at health care providers. I thank Natashe Lemos Dekker for her practical suggestions and Stefan Reinsch for sharing his analytical input and adventurous spirit. And thank you to Sjaak van der Geest for taking the time to read an early chapter draft and providing me with inspiring advice.

I am also grateful for the encouragement and inspiration I received from Seth M. Holmes at the University of California, Berkeley, who has always been generous in his appreciation of my work in the ER and has taken the time to discuss possible future developments.

Over the years, I have presented some of the book chapters and arguments in invited lectures at the Universities of Munich, Vienna, Lübeck, Warwick, Lund, Stockholm, Gothenburg, Uppsala, Aarhus, and the Ilia State in Tbilisi. I am grateful to all the seminar participants who provided me with their critical comments and sharp suggestions.

Special gratitude also goes to Danielle Mitzman for her careful and detailed proofreading of this manuscript. I wish to acknowledge my parents, Luisella and Angelo, and my brother, Alessio, for having listened to me and supported me during this project.

Last but not least, the writing process, like the emergency room, can at times be a very dark place. Thank you to my wife, Francesca Zanni, for tirelessly lighting bright sparks so that I might see my way through to the end of the tunnel.

NOTES

CHAPTER 1   URGENCY AT STAKE

1. The Italian language has three basic honorific forms that convey politeness and deference when addressing people: Signor (Mr. or sir), Signora (Mrs. or Madam), and Signorina (Miss— anyone familiar with the patriarchal bias of Italian culture will be unsurprised to discover that a marriage-neutral honorific equivalent to English's "Ms." still has not made it into Italian). These honorifics are titles and so are capitalized in Italian where, in formal contexts of address, they commonly are abbreviated as Sig., Sig.ra, and Sig.na, respectively. Because the abbreviations will be unfamiliar to most English-language readers, I have chosen not to use them in this work. Instead, I write out the words whenever I use them. But note that the words "signor," "signora," and "signorina" (in lowercase) are also used as nominals that specify gender, age, and marital status. This is how I most often use them throughout this text.

2. Throughout the monograph, the names of patients, their relatives, and the hospital staff are pseudonyms in order to safeguard their identities and protect their anonymity.

3. See, for instance, the classic work of Elliot and Vayda 1978; Dodier and Camus 1998; Vassy 2001. For more recent works, see Hillman 2014, 2016; Johannessen 2018; Buchbinder 2017; Wamsiedel 2018; Pasquini 2023a.

4. The current triage standard (2023), which uses color codes to rate urgency, was introduced in 2001 as part of a national health care agreement between the state and the twenty Italian regions directly responsible for public health care provisions (Gruppo Formazione Triage 2010).

5. See also Scheper-Hughes 1993, 2003; Biehl and Eskerod 2005; Fassin 2005, 2011; Lock and Nguyen 2010; Petryna 2013; Street 2014; Petryna and Follis 2015; Andersen 2016; McDowell 2019.

6. See Livingston 2012; Adams 2013; Street 2014; Kehr and Chabrol 2018; Solomon 2022.

7. For a complete discussion on method in hospital ethnography, see Long, Hunter, and van der Geest 2008; Wind 2008.

8. For this research I received ethical clearance from both the University of Uppsala committee and the committee of the Hospital of Emilia-Romagna, where I carried out my fieldwork. As anthropologists know, ethics is mainly a matter of everyday engagement with others. Even though I had to wear a lab coat for hygiene purposes, I always presented myself as a nonmedical researcher and took the time to explain who I was and what I was doing, making sure to disambiguate my presence in the ward as best as possible.

CHAPTER 2   A CATHEDRAL OF BIOMEDICINE

1. *Pronto soccorso* is literally translated as "ready aid" or "first aid." Throughout the book, I translate the term as "emergency room" (ER), instead of emergency department or accident and emergency, to make the text more accessible to readers who may not be familiar with hospitals and their ward divisions. The term "ER" is widely known to refer to the *pronto soccorso* department, not least due to the popular 1990s American television series of that name.

2. The relationship between the hospital and everyday social space is widely debated in hospital ethnography. A polarization exists in this debate between scholars who describe the hospital

space as an "island" under the hegemonic rule of biomedicine (e.g., Goffman 1961; Rhodes 1991) and others who instead highlight its being the "mainland," mirroring societal arrangements (e.g., van der Geest and Finkler 2004). As the anthropologists Alice Street and Simon Coleman suggest, both these scholarships overlook "hospitals' paradoxical capacity to be simultaneously bounded and permeable, both sites of social control and spaces where alternative and transgressive social orders emerge and are contested" (2012, 1). Defining hospitals as heterotopias, the authors underscore the importance of looking at the boundary making and orderings that intersect and get reshaped in the hospital (2012, 4–6; see also Brown 2012; Kehr 2018). I follow their lead by analyzing how urgency is crafted and challenged in the ER as a fluid category that results from everyday negotiations among people, technologies, spaces, and bodies.

3. Unless otherwise noted, all translations from Italian in this book are my own. "La riforma ospedaliera è un primo passo importante verso un sistema di sicurezza sociale da attuarsi nel corso di un certo periodo di tempo" (original text in Italian quoted from Cosmacini 2016, 494).

4. *The Times* article by P. Nichols and the *Economist* by N. Jucker; see Cosmacini 2016, 491.

5. "La Repubblica tutela la salute come fondamentale diritto dell'individuo e interesse della collettività, e garantisce cure gratuite agli indigenti" (Italian Constitution of 1948, art. n. XXXII).

6. This name identified a period of profound political instability and violence, conventionally starting on 12 December 1969 (the massacre of "Piazza Fontana" in Milan) and concluding on 2 August 1980 (the bomb explosion at the railway station of Bologna). The *anni di piombo* saw 140 terrorist attacks in total, with more than 160 victims and countless wounded. The vast majority of the attacks against civilians were carried out by reactionary neo-Fascist groups, followed by revolutionary anarchist and Communist factions targeting mostly journalists, functionaries, and politicians (Ginsborg 2006).

7. At the end of the 1970s, an unprecedented set of progressive reforms was introduced: the abortion law, the divorce law, the public NHS law, and law 180, a law abrogating asylums that was identified by its number and named after the psychiatrist and political activist Franco Basaglia.

8. Today 118 coexists with the general European emergency number 112 (which in Italy once connected callers to the Carabinieri, the Italian military police).

9. In Italian terminology, "emergency" and "urgency" are both listed in relation to medicine as they refer to two different, specific conditions: an emergency is a present state, and an urgency is a developing process.

10. Istituto Nazionale di Statistica (ISTAT), accessed 4 November 2019, https://www.istat.it /it/archivio/217650.

11. *Il sole 24 ore*, accessed 4 November 2019, https://www.ilsole24ore.com/art/istat-disoccu pazione-giovani-risale-401percento, in reference to ISTAT data.

12. The word "precarious" derives from "precariat," a term used to denote casual or fixed-term workers who have no guaranteed social welfare or health benefits (Han 2018). The term is largely used in the anthropological literature about Italy, where it is linked to people's diminishing economic support and worsening working conditions and to their increasing "dispossession" from the possibility of planning ahead and having a stable, secure future (Tarì and Vanni 2005; Molé 2011, 2012; Muehlebach 2012, 2013). As we will see in chapter 5, such feelings and material conditions of precarity, of invisibility, were at the center of the attention that people requested from ERs.

CHAPTER 3   TRIAGE AND ECONOMIES OF ATTENTION

1. This contact fee varies nationally according to region between €23 and €27. The ticket, as a co-payment for public medical treatment, was first introduced in 1989 in relation to diagnostic

or specialists' examinations and medication prescriptions; it was then regulated by law 537 of 1993 and subsequently applied in every region since 2001. The additional ER white-code fee of €25 was then introduced in 2011(Cosmacini 2016).

2. According to the Italian constitution: "Health is a fundamental individual right and interest of the collectivity, and Italy grants free care to the ill." Costituzione Italiana, art. XXXII, 1948, accessed 19 April 2020, https://www.senato.it/istituzione/la-costituzione/parte-i/titolo-ii/articolo-32.

3. For income assessment, the National Social Security Service (Istituto Nazionale Previdenza Sociale [INPS]) takes into consideration household composition, age, health status, bank accounts, salaries, and private properties. The INPS uses a numerical marker called ISEE (Indicatore Situazione Economica Equivalente, introduced in 1998), estimated yearly by people during tax declaration.

4. *Operatore socio-sanitario* (OSS) is difficult to translate. It is an important working figure that requires nonspecialized training of around eighteen months. The main professional mission of an OSS is to care for patients' basic needs and support nurses and doctors in their routine tasks.

5. Different colors of the scrub neckband were used to signal different positions in the ER organization: nurses, OSSes, doctors (most often also wearing a lab coat over their scrubs), or radiology technicians.

6. See Franck 2019; Citton 2017; Pedersen, Albris, and Seaver 2021.

7. As they feel that the situation of their dear ones is deeply urgent, some drive through the ambulance entry of the ER. They usually look for help to lift up their loved ones from the car and down on a hospital wheelchair.

8. At time of writing (2023), during the pandemic the staff always wore respirators, such as FFP3, FFP2, and N95. The latter were sometimes protected further with a surgical face mask on top (to help the respirators' protection last longer).

9. About SAMPLE, see Manchester Triage Group 2013; Gruppo Formazione Triage 2010.

10. The INPS is a state institution that releases and validates declarations for work injury to access welfare benefits, insurance declarations, and sick leaves.

11. According to local guidelines, the diastolic pressure needs to be equal to or over 110 and the systolic equal to or over 200 to score a full priority code, so this is a borderline case.

12. In a way, the term could be understood as close to the English "white-coat syndrome," even though the description of the "hospital effect" focuses on the anxiety produced by the setting rather than the doctor's authority.

13. The decision can also be taken before, as we saw in the case of the woman receiving the white priority code. Normally, people's blood pressure and oxygen levels at the very least are measured before deciding upon the code to be assigned.

CHAPTER 4   CHANGING TIMES

1. See Bowker and Star 2000; Street 2011b, 2012; Hull 2012.

2. One relative for each patient. In many other ERs, there is no such allowance. With his last sentence, Dr. Paolo was alluding to the fact that this rule was often a source of contestation for ER staff who preferred to deal with patients alone and often thought relatives an invasive presence.

3. Medical lab examination for assessing bacteria in the urine.

4. Normally, in Italian you address a stranger as *lei* (particularly if speaking "upward," as with doctors or other powerful professionals), which is a respectful indirect form of address. It elicits polite distance, as well as professional recognition, in this case. The *lei/tu* distance was belittling to Paolo, as it marked the generational distance with signora Gianna, as well as the existing gap between a hypothetic trusted senior doctor (*lei*) and him (*tu*), taken as just a preaching young boy.

5. Dr. Paolo had a more differential risk-based approach whose time line of progression was ill-adapted to the desire to see change and be in control as demanded by signora Gianna.

6. All physicians on duty in public care are considered as public officers capable of legal declarations.

CHAPTER 5   TRIAGE AT AN IMPASSE

1. Nurses in the *ambulatorio* are ER nurses, usually unspecialized. The possibility for a nurse "to see and treat" patients directly after triage is still controversial to some GPs as a nurse was traditionally not allowed to take full responsibility for a person or decide to discharge them. Even specialist nurses hold very few responsibilities in Italy if compared to other European Union countries like the United Kingdom, France, Spain, Germany, or Sweden. For this reason, nurses' offices are very rare in the ER and are mostly present in Tuscany at a national level.

2. In the ER where I did my fieldwork, there was neither an *ambulatorio infermieristico* nor an internal GP service. One reason for this absence was that some members of the ER staff feared that the introduction of such services would invite even more so-called nonurgent patients into the ER.

3. The referral stated a B urgency. At primary health level the priority for exam requests is rated according to a scale going from *U*, "urgente," meaning urgent; *B*, breve (a short period that usually takes around ten days); *D*, "differibile," not urgent; and *P*, "programmabile," which indicates the possibility of planning in advance for an examination with a possibly long waiting list or a specialist examination.

4. SIMEU, National Association of Italian Emergency Medicine, 2017 data on ER access.

5. Here the commercial plays with the Italian words for "ER": "Pronto Soccorso," Health Ministry of 2012, accessed 21 October 2019, https://www.youtube.com/watch?v=RT_lS5e2Ulk.

6. The original Italian reads as follows: "Il popolo è minorenne; la città è malata; ad altri spetta il compito di curare e di educare. A noi il dovere di reprimere! La repressione è il nostro vaccino. Repressione è civiltà." On the subsequent instilled desire for an authoritarian state during the coronavirus pandemic in Italy, see the work of the anthropologist Letizia Bonanno, Allegra Lab, accessed 27 April 2020, https://allegralaboratory.net/eerie-desires-for-the-authori tarian-state-covid-19-updates-from-italy/.

7. Even elderly people who did not define themselves as isolated could most often count only on their families for support—support that, due to work commitments and economic shortages, became increasingly limited. In 2018, 4 million families under stringent conditions of economic crisis had to support their elderly loved ones with no help from the state (CENSIS 2023).

8. In a sample of 1,000 people using the ER in the Emilia-Romagna region, over 62% of the calls for help came from individuals over the age of sixty-five, scoring an average of more than five accesses to the emergency service per year for each elderly person during 2017 (regional data of 2017).

9. This was the fourth Italian government led by Silvio Berlusconi (from May 2008 to November 2011).

10. This tendency started with the Bossi-Fini Law, passed in 2002 during the second Berlusconi government (which lasted from 2001 to 2005). The law was named, respectively, after Umberto Bossi, former leader of the right-wing independence party Lega Nord, and Gianfranco Fini, historical president of the Alleanza Nazionale (i.e., National Alliance) party, of clear far-right, Fascist orientation. Later on, the "Minniti Law" on migration, issued in

April 2017 and named after the then minister of internal affairs Marco Minniti, continued this trend of social exclusion. Finally, the "Decreti Sicurezza" of 2018 and 2019 (border security decrees) was introduced by the new leader of the far-right party Lega Nord, Matteo Salvini, who was minister of internal affairs at the time.

11. GPs' offices are often open only three hours per day, but they have to see all the patients who wait during those three hours, which takes much more time. The three opening hours usually alternate between mornings and afternoons during the week (GPs do not receive on weekends), in order to accommodate a wider range of people's needs. The problem is that precarious workers, working sometimes 8:00 A.M. to 8:00 P.M. or longer, often find no good time arrangement. *Corriere dell sera,* accessed 23 February 2021, https://www.corriere.it /salute/cards/medici-famiglia-doveri-diritti.

12. As calculated by AgeNaS (National Agency for Regional Health Services [Agenzia Nazio-nale per i Servizi Sanitari regionali]), the costs of contact fees and in-hospital private practice (intramoenia) for laypeople was more than €10 billion between 2012 and 2015. Quotidianos-anità.it, accessed 6 April 2020, http://www.quotidianosanita.it/allegati/allegato4360041.pdf.

13. All these in-depth examinations create images of bones and organs inside the body: through X-ray radiation (X-ray); by X-ray radiation and computer data processing (CAT scan); by strong magnetic fields and radio waves (MRI scan).

14. Quotidianosanità.it, accessed 15 June 2019, http://www.quotidianosanita.it/studi-e -analisi/articolo.php?articolo_id=74924.

15. The need to look for welfare and care, otherwise negated, in the ER can be compared to the same well-documented tendency happening in the United States where, without insur-ance coverage, one can hope for care only via the emergency service. The Italian universalistic system in this sense is dangerously evolving toward the U.S. private health care model whose unequal, socially unjust, and overly expensive outcomes are well-known (e.g. Shore 2006; Holmes et al. 2020).

CHAPTER 6   MISTRUST IN THE ER

1. Some early components of this chapter appeared in Pasquini (2023b).

2. When a medical practitioner employed by a hospital is sued, the hospital decides how, and if, to provide support by offering legal expenses to the staff member. Agenas, accessed 28 Sep-tember 2020, https://www.agenas.gov.it/denunce-sinistri-in-sanita-il-primo-report-nazionale.

3. The data are reported by the MEDMAL 12th edition report compiled by the research agency Marsh in 2021. The report is currently among the most complete sets of data regarding medical errors and lawsuits in Italy. quotidianosanita.it, "Studi de Analisi," accessed 15 March 2023, https://www.quotidianosanita.it/studi-e-analisi/articolo.php?articolo_id=86719.

4. The vast scholarship about trust comprises widely different works, like the work on social relations by the sociologist Diego Gambetta (1990) and the more conservative comparison of state institutions led by scholars like the political theorist Francis Fukuyama (1996). But as the anthropologist Florian Mühlfried (2019) points out, studies on trust share a general ten-dency to disregard mistrust as a real topic of inquiry and consider it as just a lack of trust. See also "The Problem of Trust" by Seligman (2000); "Trust in Society" by Cook (2003); "Trust and Trustworthiness" and simply "Trust" by Hardin (2002); "Trust, Ethics and Human Rea-son" by Lagerspetz et al. (2015; cf. Möllering 2005).

5. Anthropologists studying epidemic outbreaks, particularly HIV and Ebola, have also par-tially addressed the effects of mistrust. For instance, the physician and anthropologist Paul Farmer (2006) addressed the social effects of suspicions and rumors, which can be taken as expressions of mistrust, by describing the diverse colonial and power relations that guided

their spread during the HIV outbreak in Haiti, creating what he calls "geographies of blame" (see also Abramowitz 2017, 427).

6. *Corriere della sera*, accessed 15 February 2021, https://www.corriere.it/cronache/18_luglio _20/lugo-infermiera-killer.

7. *La Repubblica*, "Archivio," accessed 15 February 2021, https://ricerca.repubblica.it/repub blica/archivio.

8. *La Repubblica*, "Archivio."

9. Report on insurance, compensations, and lawsuits for malpractice and medical errors: IVASS, 2018, accessed 15 February 2021, https://www.ivass.it/pubblicazioni-e-statistiche.

10. Self-diagnosis played a foundational role in patient-staff relationships. The anthropologist Sylvie Fainzang's work on self-medication in France suggests that when people consult Internet forums and websites, "sociality" emerges (2016). United around shared concerns, people go online (1) seeking information about symptoms, medicaments, and their effects and (2) advocating or opposing the use of certain drugs, therefore contributing to Internet-based discussions.

11. The Italian CENSIS (Centro Studi Investimenti Sociali [Center for Social Studies and Investments]) describes the situation of women's employment in Italy as dramatic, the absolute worst in Europe with regard to precariousness of contracts and number of work positions held (https://www.censis.it/sicurezza-e-cittadinanza/donne-lontane-dagli-uomini-e-lontane -dall%E2%80%99europa-il-gender-gap-nel-lavoro, accessed 7 May 2020). Now, during, and after the COVID-19 pandemic, women's working conditions have worsened further since no arrangements were/have been made to face the need of many to combine care work with the demands of a collapsing neoliberal job market. *La Repubblica*, accessed 7 May 2020, https://www.repubblica.it/solidarieta/diritti.

CHAPTER 7   VIOLENCE AND ITS CONSEQUENCES

1. Some early components of this chapter appeared in Pasquini (2023a).

2. An example of such cases, linked to criminal organizations, was the devastation of the ER of the San Pellegrino Hospital in Naples by the relatives of a fifteen-year-old who died during an attempted robbery. See *la Repubblica*, "Napoli," accessed 3 July 2020, https: //napoli. repubblica.it/cronaca/2020/03/03/news.

3. NURSID campaign, 16 January 2020, https://www.dire.it/16-01-2020/410852-video-eva -grimaldi-testimonial.

4. There is plenty more international evidence of the escalation of violence against ER workers. See, for instance, Jiao et al. 2015 (China).

5. *Corriere della sera*, 3 July 2020, https://www.corriere.it/politica/3/7/2020. This attempt was met with open hostility by many national medical and nursing organizations. By the motto "Io curo, non restringo, non denuncio" (I treat [everyone], I do not restrain, I do not report [illegal migrants]), professionals retorted that increasing police and Carabinieri (military police) presence in the ER would lead to an escalation, rather than a de-escalation, of violence. The proposal never went through.

6. See Das and Poole 2004; Das 2006; Ticktin 2011; Giordano 2014; Holmes et al. 2020.

7. Such a pose and resolute military walking can be interpreted as deliberately inspired by the stereotypical masculinities of the Italian Fascist period of the 1920s.

8. State attorney investigations into violent happenings rested heavily on days of continued symptoms used as a benchmark measure for the gravity of physical injuries. Back in 2018, the Italian law provided for automatic legal proceedings only if wounds led to at least thirty days of continued symptoms. This practically meant broken bones, diffused third-degree burns,

copious internal bleeding, or organ failure. Such regulations were ill-adapted to the documented widespread incidence of gender violence in Italy, leaving the responsibility for any legal proceedings to women alone and often failing to protect their safety before their injuries escalated to a desperate level after outbursts of violence.

CONCLUSIONS

1. The man had interstitial bilateral pneumonia (a condition that would become recognized as typical of the pneumonia caused by the novel coronavirus Sars-CoV-2), and he did not respond to any antibiotic therapy.

2. Istituto Superiore di Sanità, accessed 20 March 2021, https://www.epicentro.iss.it /coronavirus/sars-cov-2-decessi-italia#2 accessed 20/3/2021.

3. From the original Italian: "La Repubblica tutela la salute come fondamentale diritto dell'individuo e interesse della collettività, e garantisce cure gratuite agli indigenti" (Costituzione della Repubblica Italiana of 1948, art. n XXXII, para. 1).

4. The report is released annually by the national Center for Social Studies and Investments, Censis (Centro Studi e Investimenti Sociali), in collaboration with RBM, a private health insurance firm. *Sanità informazione*, accessed 23 March 2021, https://www.sanitainformazione .it/wp-content/uploads/2021/02/IX-Rapporto-sulla-Sanita-Pubblica-Privata-e-Intermediata .pdf.

5. This phenomenon was particularly strong in Lombardy, where 40% of all health care services are privately owned. *New York Times*, accessed 3 March 2021, https://www.nytimes .com/2020/11/19/business/lombardy-italy-coronavirus-doctors.html; *Guardian*, accessed 19 March 2021, https://www.theguardian.com/commentisfree/ 2020/dec/24/covid-crisis -privatisation-democracy-outsourcing.

REFERENCES

Aacharya, Ramesh P., Chris Gastmans, and Yvonne Denier. 2011. "Emergency Department Triage: An Ethical Analysis." *BMC Emergency Medicine* 11 (October): 16. https://doi.org /10.1186/1471-227X-11-16.

Abramowitz, Sharon. 2017. "Epidemics (Especially Ebola)." *Annual Review of Anthropology* 46 (1): 421–445. https://doi.org/10.1146/annurev-anthro-102116-041616.

Adams, Vincanne. 2013. *Markets of Sorrow, Labors of Faith: New Orleans in the Wake of Katrina.* Durham, NC: Duke University Press.

Adams, Vincanne, Michelle Murphy, and Adele E. Clarke. 2009. "Anticipation: Technoscience, Life, Affect, Temporality." *Subjectivity* 28 (1): 246–265. https://doi.org/10.1057/sub .2009.18.Akshay Khanna, Ian Harper, and Tobias Kelly. 2015. *The Clinic and the Court.* 1st ed. Cambridge: Cambridge University Press.

Alfieri, Chiara, Marc Egrot, Alice Desclaux, and Kelley Sams. 2022. "Recognising Italy's Mistakes in the Public Health Response to COVID-19." *Lancet* 399 (10322): 357–358. https://doi.org/10.1016/S0140-6736(21)02805-1.

Allison, Anne. 2012. "Ordinary Refugees: Social Precarity and Soul in 21st Century Japan." *Anthropological Quarterly* 85 (2): 345–370.

———. 2013. *Precarious Japan.* Durham, NC: Duke University Press.

Ameri, Marta, Paolo Cremonesi, and Marcello Montefiori. 2011. "Pronto soccorso e spesa sanitaria regionale." *Politiche sanitarie* 12 (4): 190–198.

Andersen, Barbara. 2016. "Temporal Circuits and Social Triage in a Papua New Guinean Clinic." *Critique of Anthropology* 36 (1): 13–26.

Armocida, Benedetta, Beatrice Formenti, Silvia Ussai, Francesca Palestra, and Eduardo Missoni. 2020. "The Italian Health System and the COVID-19 Challenge." *Lancet Public Health* 5 (5): e253. https://doi.org/10.1016/S2468-2667(20)30074-8.

Auyero, Javier. 2012. *Patients of the State: The Politics of Waiting in Argentina.* Durham, NC: Duke University Press.

Beckett, Greg. 2013. "The Politics of Emergency." *Reviews in Anthropology* 42 (2): 85–101. https://doi.org/10.1080/00938157.2013.788348.

Berlinger, Nancy. 2016. *Are Workarounds Ethical? Managing Moral Problems in Health Care Systems.* Oxford: Oxford University Press.

Biehl, João Guilherme, and Torben Eskerod. 2005. *Vita: Life in a Zone of Social Abandonment.* Berkeley: University of California Press.

Biehl, João Guilherme, Byron Good, and Arthur Kleinman, eds. 2007. *Subjectivity: Ethnographic Investigations.* 1st ed. Berkeley: University of California Press.

Blackman, Lisa, John Cromby, Derek Hook, Dimitris Papadopoulos, and Valerie Walkerdine. 2008. "Creating Subjectivities." *Subjectivity* 22 (1): 1–27. https://doi.org/10.1057/sub.2008.8.

Bodini, Chiara, and Ivo Quaranta. 2021. "COVID-19 in Italy: A New Culture of Healthcare for Future Preparedness." In *Viral Loads,* edited by Lenore Manderson, Nancy J. Burke, and Ayo Wahlberg, 443–455. Anthropologies of Urgency in the Time of COVID-19. London: University College London Press. https://www.jstor.org/stable/j.ctv1j13zb3.29.

Bourdieu, Pierre. 1977. *Outline of a Theory of Practice.* Translated by Richard Nice. 1st ed. Cambridge: Cambridge University Press.

Bowker, Geoffrey C., and Susan Leigh Star. 2000. *Sorting Things Out: Classification and Its Consequences*. 1st ed. Cambridge, MA: MIT Press.

Brown, Hannah. 2012. "Hospital Domestics: Care Work in a Kenyan Hospital." *Space and Culture* 15 (1): 18–30. https://doi.org/10.1177/1206331211426056.

Brown, Patrick R. 2008. "Trusting in the New NHS: Instrumental versus Communicative Action." *Sociology of Health and Illness* 30 (3): 349–363. https://doi.org/10.1111/j.1467-9566.2007.01065.x.

Bruun, Maja Hojer, Astrid Oberborbeck Andersen, and Adrienne Mannov. 2020. "Infrastructures of Trust and Distrust: The Politics and Ethics of Emerging Cryptographic Technologies." *Anthropology Today* 36 (2): 13–17.

Buchbinder, Mara. 2017. "Keeping Out and Getting In: Reframing Emergency Department Gatekeeping as Structural Competence." *Sociology of Health and Illness* 39 (7): 1166–1179. https://doi.org/10.1111/1467-9566.12566.

Butler, Judith. 2006. *Precarious Life: The Powers of Mourning and Violence*. Reprint ed. New York: Verso.

Caduff, Carlo. 2015. *The Pandemic Perhaps: Dramatic Events in a Public Culture of Danger*. 1st ed. Berkeley: University of California Press.

Canguilhem, Georges. 1988. "Le statut épistémologique de la médecine." *History and Philosophy of the Life Sciences* 10:15–29.

Capello, Carlo. 2020. *Ai margini del lavoro: Un'antropologia della disoccupazione a Torino*. Verona: Ombre Corte.

Carey, Matthew. 2017. *Mistrust: An Ethnographic Theory*. Chicago: University of Chiago Press.

CENSIS. 2023. *57° Rapporto Sulla Situazione Sociale Del Paese 2023*. 1st ed. Milan: Franco Angeli.

Chambliss, Daniel F. 1996. *Beyond Caring: Hospitals, Nurses, and the Social Organization of Ethics*. Chicago: University of Chicago Press.

Citton, Yves. 2016. *The Ecology of Attention*. Translated by Barnaby Norman. Cambridge: Polity Press.

Comodo, Nicola, and Gavino Maciocco. 2011. *Igiene e sanità pubblica: Manuale per le professioni sanitarie*. Rome: Carocci.

Conrad, Peter. 2007. *The Medicalization of Society: On the Transformation of Human Conditions into Treatable Disorders*. 1st ed. Baltimore: Johns Hopkins University Press.

Cook, Joanna, and Catherine Trundle. 2020. "Unsettled Care: Temporality, Subjectivity, and the Uneasy Ethics of Care." *Anthropology and Humanism* 45 (2): 178–183. https://doi.org/10.1111/anhu.12308.

Cook, Karen. 2003. *Trust in Society*. New York: Russell Sage Foundation.

Cosmacini, Giorgio. 2016. *Storia della medicina e della sanità in Italia: Dalla peste nera ai giorni nostri*. Bari, Italy: Laterza.

Costa, Giuseppe, Maurizio Bassi, Gian Franco Gensini, Michele Marra, and Anna Lisa Nicelli. 2016. *L'equità nella salute in Italia: Secondo rapporto sulle disuguaglianze sociali in sanità*. Milan: Franco Angeli.

Csordas, Thomas J. 1990. "Embodiment as a Paradigm for Anthropology." *Ethos* 18 (1): 5–47.

———. 1993. "Somatic Modes of Attention." *Cultural Anthropology* 8 (2): 135–156.

Das, Veena. 2006. *Life and Words: Violence and the Descent into the Ordinary*. 1st ed. Berkeley: University of California Press.

———. 2008. "Violence, Gender, and Subjectivity." *Annual Review of Anthropology* 37 (1): 283–299. https://doi.org/10.1146/annurev.anthro.36.081406.094430.

Das, Veena, and Deborah Poole. 2004. *Anthropology in the Margins of the State*. Santa Fe: School for Advanced Research.

Derber, Charles. 2000. *The Pursuit of Attention: Power and Ego in Everyday Life*. 2nd ed6. New York: Oxford University Press.

Di Somma, Salvatore, Lorenzo Paladino, Louella Vaughan, Irene Lalle, Laura Magrini, and Massimo Magnanti. 2015. "Overcrowding in Emergency Department: An International Issue." *Internal and Emergency Medicine* 10 (2): 171–175. https://doi.org/10.1007/s11739-014-1154-8.

Dodier, Nicholas, and Agnès Camus. 1998. "Openness and Specialisation: Dealing with Patients in a Hospital Emergency Service." *Sociology of Health & Illness* 20 (4): 413–444. https://doi.org/10.1111/1467-9566.00109.

Dongen, Els Van. 2002. "Theatres of the Lie: 'Crazy' Deception and Lying as Drama." *Anthropology and Medicine* 9 (2): 135–151. https://doi.org/10.1080/1364847022000029714.

———. 2003. *Walking Stories: An Oddnography of Mad People's Work with Culture*. Amsterdam: Rozenberg.

Dongen, Els Van, and Sylvie Fainzang, eds. 2005. *Lying and Illness: Power and Performance*. Amsterdam: Het Spinhuis.

Doupe, Malcolm B., Wes Palatnick, Suzanne Day, Dan Chateau, Ruth-Ann Soodeen, Charles Burchill, and Shelley Derksen. 2012. "Frequent Users of Emergency Departments: Developing Standard Definitions and Defining Prominent Risk Factors." *Annals of Emergency Medicine* 60 (1): 24–32. https://doi.org/10.1016/j.annemergmed.2011.11.036.

Edwards, Phil. 2005. "The Berlusconi Anomaly: Populism and Patrimony in Italy's Long Transition." *South European Society and Politics* 10 (2): 225–243. https://doi.org/10.1080/136087 40500134945.

Elliott, Marshall J., and Eugene Vayda. 1978. "Characteristics of Emergency Department Users." *Canadian Journal of Public Health/Revue Canadienne de Sante'e Publique* 69 (3): 233–238.

Fainzang, Sylvie. 2015. *An Anthropology of Lying: Information in the Doctor-Patient Relationship*. 1st ed. London: Routledge.

———. 2016. *Self-Medication and Society: Mirages of Autonomy*. 1st ed. London: Routledge.

Farmer, Paul. 2004. "An Anthropology of Structural Violence." *Current Anthropology* 45 (3): 305–325. https://doi.org/10.1086/382250.

———. 2006. *AIDS and Accusation: Haiti and the Geography of Blame*. 1st ed. Berkeley: University of California Press. Updated with a new preface.

Fassin, Didier. 2005. "Compassion and Repression: The Moral Economy of Immigration Policies in France." *Cultural Anthropology* 20 (3): 362–387. https://doi.org/10.1525/can.2005.20.3.362.

———. 2011a. *Humanitarian Reason: A Moral History of the Present*. Translated by Rachel Gomme. Berkeley: University of California Press.

———. 2011b. "Policing Borders, Producing Boundaries: The Governmentality of Immigration in Dark Times." *Annual Review of Anthropology* 40 (1): 213–226. https://doi.org/10 .1146/annurev-anthro-081309-145847.

———. 2015. *At the Heart of the State: The Moral World of Institutions*. London: Pluto Press.

Fassin, Didier, and Mariella Pandolfi. 2010. *Contemporary States of Emergency: The Politics of Military and Humanitarian Interventions*. Cambridge, MA: Zone Books.

Ferns, Terry. 2006. "Under-Reporting of Violent Incidents against Nursing Staff." *Nursing Standard* (Great Britain) 20 (40): 41–45. https://doi.org/10.7748/ns2006.06.20.40.41.c4178.

Foucault, Michel. 1988. *Power/Knowledge: Selected Interviews and Other Writings, 1972–1977*. New York: Vintage Books.

———. 1991a. *Discipline and Punish: The Birth of the Prison*. Translated by Alan Sheridan. London: Penguin.

———. 1991b. "Governmentality." In *The Foucault Effects: Studies in Governmentality*, edited by G. Burchell, C. Gordon, and P. Miller, 87–104. London: Harvester Wheatsheaf.

———. 1994. *The Birth of the Clinic*. 3rd ed. London: Routledge.

————. 1998. *The History of Sexuality*. Vol. 1, *The Will to Knowledge*. Translated by Robert Hurley. New ed. London: Penguin.

————. 2004. *"Society Must Be Defended": Lectures at the Collège de France, 1975–76*. Edited by Mauro Bertani. Translated by David Macey. London: Penguin.

Franck, Georg. 2019. "The Economy of Attention." *Journal of Sociology* 55 (1): 8–19. https://doi.org/10.1177/1440783318811778.

Fukuyama, Francis. 1996. *Trust: The Social Virtues and the Creation of Prosperity: Human Nature and the Reconstitution of Social Order*. New York: Free Press.

Gacki-Smith, Jessica, Altair M. Juarez, Lara Boyett, Cathy Homeyer, Linda Robinson, and Susan L. MacLean. 2010. "Violence against Nurses Working in US Emergency Departments." *Journal of Healthcare Protection Management: Publication of the International Association for Hospital Security* 26 (1): 81–99.

Gama e Colombo, Daniel. 2010. "Closing the Gap in a Generation: Health Equity through Action on the Social Determinants of Health. Final Report of the Commission on Social Determinants of Health." *Revista de direito sanitário* 10 (3): 253. https://doi.org/10.11606/issn.2316-9044.v10i3p253-266.

Gambetta, Diego. 1990. *Trust: Making and Breaking Cooperative Relations*. Reprint, Oxford: Blackwell.

Garcia, Angela. 2010. *The Pastoral Clinic: Addiction and Dispossession along the Rio Grande*. 1st ed. Berkeley: University of California Press.

Geest, Sjaak van der, and Kaja Finkler. 2004. "Hospital Ethnography: Introduction." *Social Science and Medicine (1982)* 59 (10): 1995–2001.

Gibson, Diana. 2004. "The Gaps in the Gaze in South African Hospitals." *Social Science and Medicine (1982)* 59 (10): 2013–2024.

Gille, Felix, Sarah Smith, and Nicholas Mays. 2015. "Why Public Trust in Health Care Systems Matters and Deserves Greater Research Attention." *Journal of Health Services Research and Policy* 20 (1): 62–64.

Gilson, Lucy. 2006. "Trust in Health Care: Theoretical Perspectives and Research Needs." *Journal of Health Organization and Management* 20 (5): 359–375.

Ginsborg, Paul. 2006. *Storia d'Italia dal dopoguerra a oggi*. Translated by Sandro Perini and Marcello Flores. 2nd ed. Turin: Einaudi.

Giordano, Cristiana. 2014. *Migrants in Translation*. Berkeley: University of California Press.

Goffman, Erving. 1961. *Asylums: Essays on the Social Situation of Mental Patients and Other Inmates*. Reprint, New York: Anchor Books.

Greco, Cinzia. 2019. "Moving for Cures: Breast Cancer and Mobility in Italy." *Medical Anthropology* 38 (4): 384–398. https://doi.org/10.1080/01459740.2019.1592171.

Grover, Casey A., and Reb J. H. Close. 2009. "Frequent Users of the Emergency Department: Risky Business." *Western Journal of Emergency Medicine* 10 (3): 193–194.

Gruppo Formazione Triage (Triage Training Group). 2010. *Triage infermieristico*. 3rd ed. Milan: McGraw Hill Education.

Habermas, Juergen. 1975. *Legitimation Crisis*. Translated by Thomas McCarthy. Boston: Beacon Press.

Hadolt, Bernhard, and Anita Hardon. 2017. *Emerging Socialities and Subjectivities in Twenty-First-Century Healthcare*. 1st ed. Amsterdam: Amsterdam University Press.

Han, Clara. 2011. "Symptoms of Another Life: Time, Possibility, and Domestic Relations in Chile's Credit Economy." *Cultural Anthropology* 26 (1): 7–32. https://doi.org/10.1111/j.1548-1360.2010.01078.x.

————. 2012. *Life in Debt: Times of Care and Violence in Neoliberal Chile*. Berkeley: University of California Press.

———. 2018. "Precarity, Precariousness, and Vulnerability." *Annual Review of Anthropology* 47 (1): 331–343. https://doi.org/10.1146/annurev-anthro-102116-041644.

Hardin, Russell. 2002. *Trust and Trustworthiness*. New York: Russell Sage Foundation.

Herzfeld, Michael. 1980. "Honour and Shame: Problems in the Comparative Analysis of Moral Systems." *Man* 15 (2): 339–351. https://doi.org/10.2307/2801675.

———. 2009. *Evicted from Eternity: The Restructuring of Modern Rome*. Chicago: University of Chicago Press.

Hillman, Alexandra. 2014. "'Why Must I Wait?' The Performance of Legitimacy in a Hospital Emergency Department." *Sociology of Health and Illness* 36 (4): 485–499. https://doi.org/10.1111/1467-9566.12072.

———. 2016. "Institutions of Care, Moral Proximity and Demoralisation: The Case of the Emergency Department." *Social Theory and Health* (Basingstoke) 14 (1): 66–87. http://dx.doi.org.ezproxy.its.uu.se/10.1057/sth.2015.10.

Hodge, Alister N., and Andrea P. Marshall. 2007. "Violence and Aggression in the Emergency Department: A Critical Care Perspective." *Australian Critical Care: Official Journal of the Confederation of Australian Critical Care Nurses* 20 (2): 61–67. https://doi.org/10.1016/j.aucc.2007.03.001.

Holmes, Seth M., Helena Hansen, Angela Jenks, Scott D. Stonington, Michelle Morse, Jeremy A. Greene, Keith A. Wailoo, Michael G. Marmot, and Paul Farmer. 2020. "Misdiagnosis, Mistreatment, and Harm—When Medical Care Ignores Social Forces." *New England Journal of Medicine* 382 (12): 1083–1086. https://doi.org/10.1056/NEJMp1916269.

Horton, Richard. 2005. "The Neglected Epidemic of Chronic Disease." *Lancet* 366 (9496): 1514. https://doi.org/10.1016/S0140-6736(05)67454-5.

Hull, Elizabeth. 2012. "Paperwork and the Contradictions of Accountability in a South African Hospital." *Journal of the Royal Anthropological Institute* 18 (3): 613–632. https://doi.org/10.1111/j.1467-9655.2012.01779.x.

Husserl, Edmund. 1962. *Ideas: General Introduction to Pure Phenomenology*. New York: Collier Books.

Hyde, Sandra Teresa, and Laurie Denyer Willis. 2020. "Balancing the Quotidian: Precarity, Care and Pace in Anthropology's Storytelling." *Medical Anthropology* 39 (4): 297–304. https://doi.org/10.1080/01459740.2020.1739673.

Inda, Jonathan Xavier, ed. 2005. *Anthropologies of Modernity: Foucault, Governmentality, and Life Politics*. Oxford: Blackwell.

Iserson, Kenneth V., and John C. Moskop. 2007. "Triage in Medicine." Part I, "Concept, History, and Types." *Annals of Emergency Medicine* 49 (3): 275–281. https://doi.org/10.1016/j.annemergmed.2006.05.019.

James, William. 1950. *The Principles of Psychology*. Vol. 1. Reprint, New York: Dover.

Jeong, Jong-min. 2020. "Rethinking Repetition in Dementia through a Cartographic Ethnography of Subjectivity." *Medicine Anthropology Theory* 7 (1). https://doi.org/10.17157/mat.7.1.644.

Jiao, Mingli, Ning Ning, Ye Li, Lijun Gao, Yu Cui, Hong Sun, Zheng Kang, Libo Liang, Qunhong Wu, and Yanhua Hao. 2015. "Workplace Violence against Nurses in Chinese Hospitals: A Cross-Sectional Survey." *BMJ Open* 5 (3): e006719. https://doi.org/10.1136/bmjopen-2014-006719.

Johannessen, Lars E. F. 2018. "Narratives and Gatekeeping: Making Sense of Triage Nurses' Practice." *Sociology of Health and Illness* 40 (5): 892–906. https://doi.org/10.1111/1467-9566.12732.

———. 2019. "The Commensuration of Pain: How Nurses Transform Subjective Experience into Objective Numbers." *Social Science and Medicine* 233 (July): 38–46. https://doi.org/10.1016/j.socscimed.2019.05.042.

Kaufman, Sharon R. 2006. *And a Time to Die: How American Hospitals Shape the End of Life.* 1st ed. Chicago: University of Chicago Press.

———. 2015. *Ordinary Medicine: Extraordinary Treatments, Longer Lives, and Where to Draw the Line.* 1st ed. Durham, NC: Duke University Press.

Kehr, Janina. 2018. "Colonial Hauntings: Migrant Care in a French Hospital." *Medical Anthropology* 37 (8): 659–673. https://doi.org/10.1080/01459740.2018.1518982.

Kehr, Janina, and Fanny Chabrol. 2018. "L'hôpital." *Anthropologie & Santé. Revue internationale francophone d'anthropologie de la santé,* no. 16 (May). http://journals.openedition.org /anthropologiesante/2997.

Kipnis, Andrew B. 2008. "Audit Cultures: Neoliberal Governmentality, Socialist Legacy, or Technologies of Governing?" *American Ethnologist* 35 (2): 275–289.

Klaver, Klaartje, and Andries Baart. 2011. "Attentive Care in a Hospital." *Medische Antropologie* 23 (2): 309–324.

Kleinman, A., and S. van der Geest. 2009. "'Care' in Health Care: Remaking the Moral World of Medicine." *Medische antropologie* 21:159–168. https://dare.uva.nl/search?identifier=b7b9 71cd-7cfd-445b-937a-1cccd7494254.

Krause, Elizabeth L. 2009. *Unraveled: A Weaver's Tale of Life Gone Modern.* Berkeley: University of California Press.

Kulick, Don, and Jens Rydström. 2015. *Loneliness and Its Opposite: Sex, Disability, and the Ethics of Engagement.* Durham, NC: Duke University Press.

Lachenal, Guillaume, Céline Lefève, and Vinh-Kim Nguyen. 2014. *La médecine du tri. Histoire, éthique, anthropologie.* Paris: Presses Universitaires de France.

Lagerspetz, Olli, Simon Kirchin, and Thom Brooks. 2015. *Trust, Ethics and Human Reason.* London: Bloomsbury Academic.

Larkin, Brian. 2013. "The Politics and Poetics of Infrastructure." *Annual Review of Anthropology* 42 (1): 327–343. https://doi.org/10.1146/annurev-anthro-092412-155522.

Latour, Bruno. 2007. *Reassembling the Social: An Introduction to Actor-Network-Theory.* Oxford: Oxford University Press.

Livingston, Julie. 2012. *Improvising Medicine: An African Oncology Ward in an Emerging Cancer Epidemic.* 1st ed. Durham, NC: Duke University Press.

Lock, Margaret. 2002. "Inventing a New Death and Making It Believable." *Anthropology and Medicine* 9 (2): 97–115. https://doi.org/10.1080/1364847022000029705.

———. 2017. "Recovering the Body." *Annual Review of Anthropology* 46 (1): 1–14. https://doi .org/10.1146/annurev-anthro-102116-041253.

Lock, Margaret, and Nguyen Vinh-Kim. 2010. *An Anthropology of Biomedicine.* 1st ed. John Wiley and Sons. Chichester, UK: Wiley-Blackwell.

Long, Debbi, Cynthia Hunter, and Sjaak van der Geest. 2008. "When the Field Is a Ward or a Clinic: Hospital Ethnography." *Anthropology and Medicine* 15 (2): 71–78. https://doi.org /10.1080/13648470802121844.

Maciocco, Gavino 2019. *Cure primarie e servizi territoriali: Esperienze nazionali e internazionali.* Rome: Carocci.

Manchester Triage Group. 2013. *Emergency Triage.* 3rd ed. London: BMJ Books.

Manderson, Lenore, Nancy J. Burke, and Ayo Wahlberg. 2021. *Viral Loads: Anthropologies of Urgency in the Time of COVID-19.* London: University College London Press.

Manderson, Lenore, and Carolyn Smith-Morris, eds. 2010. *Chronic Conditions, Fluid States: Chronicity and the Anthropology of Illness.* New Brunswick, NJ: Rutgers University Press. http://ebookcentral.proquest.com/lib/uu/detail.action?docID=864876.

Manderson, Lenore, and Ayo Wahlberg. 2020. "Chronic Living in a Communicable World." *Medical Anthropology* 39 (5): 428–439.

Marsland, Rebecca, and Ruth Prince. 2012. "What Is Life Worth? Exploring Biomedical Interventions, Survival, and the Politics of Life." *Medical Anthropology Quarterly* 26 (4): 453–469. https://doi.org/10.1111/maq.12001.

Martin, Emily. 1995. *Flexible Bodies: Tracking Immunity in American Culture—from the Days of Polio to the Age of AIDS.* New ed. Boston: Beacon Press.

Martin, Luther H., Huck Gutman, and Patrick H. Hutton. 1998. *Technologies of the Self: A Seminar with Michel Foucault.* Amherst: University of Massachusetts Press.

Mattingly, Cheryl. 1994. "The Concept of Therapeutic 'Emplotment.'" *Social Science and Medicine* 38 (6): 811–822. https://doi.org/10.1016/0277-9536(94)90153.

———. 1998. "In Search of the Good: Narrative Reasoning in Clinical Practice." *Medical Anthropology Quarterly* 12 (3): 273–297.

———. 2009. *Healing Dramas and Clinical Plots: The Narrative Structure of Experience.* Cambridge: Cambridge University Press.

———. 2019. "Waiting: Anticipation and Episodic Time." *Cambridge Journal of Anthropology* 37 (1): 17–31. https://doi.org/10.3167/cja.2019.370103.

Mbembe, Achille. 2019. *Necropolitics.* Translated by Steven Corcoran. Durham, NC: Duke University Press.

McDowell, Andrew. 2019. "Dr. Ram's Triage." *Medicine Anthropology Theory* 6 (4). https://doi.org/10.17157/mat.6.4.735.

McHale, Philip, Sara Wood, Karen Hughes, Mark A. Bellis, Ulf Demnitz, and Sacha Wyke. 2013. "Who Uses Emergency Departments Inappropriately and When—a National Cross-Sectional Study Using a Monitoring Data System." *BMC Medicine* 11 (1): 258. https://doi.org/10.1186/1741-7015-11-258.

Meng, Zhaolin, Wen Hui, Yuanyi Cai, Jiazhou Liu, and Huazhang Wu. 2020. "The Effects of DRGs-Based Payment Compared with Cost-Based Payment on Inpatient Healthcare Utilization: A Systematic Review and Meta-Analysis." *Health Policy* (Amsterdam) 124 (4): 359–367. https://doi.org/10.1016/j.healthpol.2020.01.007.

Merleau-Ponty, Maurice. 2013. *Phenomenology of Perception.* Edited by Taylor Carman. Translated by Donald Landes. 1st ed. Abingdon, England: Routledge.

Mol, Annemarie. 2002. *The Body Multiple: Ontology in Medical Practice.* Durham, NC: Duke University Press.

———. 2008. *The Logic of Care: Health and the Problem of Patient Choice.* 1st ed. London: Routledge.

Mol, Annemarie, Ingunn Moser, and Jeannette Pols, eds. 2010. *Care in Practice: On Tinkering in Clinics, Homes and Farms.* 1st ed. Bielefeld, Germany: Transcript-Verlag.

Molé, Noelle J. 2011. *Labor Disorders in Neoliberal Italy: Mobbing, Well-Being, and the Workplace.* Bloomington: Indiana University Press.

———. 2012. "Hauntings of Solidarity in Post-Fordist Italy." *Anthropological Quarterly* 85 (2): 371–396.

———. 2013. "Trusted Puppets, Tarnished Politicians: Humor and Cynicism in Berlusconi's Italy." *American Ethnologist* 40 (2): 288–299. https://doi.org/10.1111/amet.12021.

Möllering, Guido. 2005. "Understanding Trust from the Perspective of Sociological Neoinstitutionalism: The Interplay of Institutions and Agency." SSRN Scholarly Paper ID 1456838. Rochester, NY: Social Science Research Network. https://doi.org/10.2139/ssrn.1456838.

Moskop, John C., and Kenneth V. Iserson. 2007. "Triage in Medicine." Part II, "Underlying Values and Principles." *Annals of Emergency Medicine* 49 (3): 282–287. https://doi.org/10.1016/j.annemergmed.2006.07.012.

Muehlebach, Andrea. 2012. *The Moral Neoliberal: Welfare and Citizenship in Italy.* Chicago: University of Chicago Press.

———. 2013. "On Precariousness and the Ethical Imagination: The Year 2012 in Sociocultural Anthropology." *American Anthropologist* 115 (2): 297–311. https://doi.org/10.1111/aman.12011.

Mühlfried, Florian, ed. 2017. *Mistrust: Ethnographic Approximations*. Bielefeld, Germany: Transcript-Verlag.

———. 2019. *Mistrust: A Global Perspective*. London: Palgrave Pivot. https://doi.org/10.1007/978-3-030-11470-1.

Mulla, Sameena. 2014. *The Violence of Care: Rape Victims, Forensic Nurses, and Sexual Assault Intervention*. New York: New York University Press.

Napier, A. David, Clyde Ancarno, Beverley Butler, Joseph Calabrese, Angel Chater, Helen Chatterjee, François Guesnet, et al. 2014. "Culture and Health." *Lancet* 384 (9954): 1607–1639. https://doi.org/10.1016/S0140-6736(14)61603-2.

Nguyen, Vinh-Kim. 2010. *The Republic of Therapy: Triage and Sovereignty in West Africa's Time of AIDS*. 1st ed. Durham, NC: Duke University Press.

OECD Health Spending. (n.d.). "OECD Data Indicators." Accessed 28 December 2024. https://www.oecd.org/en/data/indicators/health-spending.html?oecdcontrol-00b22b2429-var3=2018.

O'Keeffe, Colin, Suzanne Mason, Richard Jacques, and Jon Nicholl. 2018. "Characterising Non-urgent Users of the Emergency Department (ED): A Retrospective Analysis of Routine ED Data." *PLOS ONE* 13 (2): e0192855. https://doi.org/10.1371/journal.pone.0192855.

Ong, Aihwa, and Stephen J. Collier, eds. 2004. *Global Assemblages: Technology, Politics, and Ethics as Anthropological Problems*. 1st ed. Malden, MA: Wiley-Blackwell.

Osservatorio Nazionale. 2018. "Rapporto Osservasalute 2018/Osservatorio sulla Salute." Accessed 6 February 2021. https://www.osservatoriosullasalute.it/osservasalute/rapporto-osservatorio-2018.

Pandolfi, Mariella. 2003. "Contract of Mutual (In)Difference: Government and the Humanitarian Apparatus in Contemporary Albania and Kosovo." *Indiana Journal of Global Legal Studies* 10 (1): 369–381. https://www.repository.law.indiana.edu/ijgls/vol10/iss1/13.

Pasquini, Mirko. 2023a. "Like Ticking Time Bombs: Improvising Structural Competency to 'Defuse' the Exploding of Violence against Emergency Care Workers in Italy." *Global Public Health* 0 (0): 1–12. https://doi.org/10.1080/17441692.2022.2141291.

———. 2023b. "Mistrustful Dependency: Mistrust as Risk-Management in an Italian Emergency Department." *Medical Anthropology: Cross-Cultural Studies in Health and Illness* 42 (6): 579–592.

———. 2024. "The Sound of the Absurd: Learning to Listen in the Emergency Room (ER)." In *Stop Making Sense: Anthropology of the Absurd* (blog), edited by Carline Kopft, Ståle Wig, and Chaterine Alexander. Allegra Lab: Anthropology for Radical Optimism.

Pedersen, Line Hjøllund, Ayo Wahlberg, Marie Cordt, Kjeld Schmiegelow, Susanne Oksbjerg Dalton, and Hanne Bækgaard Larsen. 2020. "Parent's Perspectives of the Pathway to Diagnosis of Childhood Cancer: A Matter of Diagnostic Triage." *BMC Health Services Research* 20 (1): 969. https://doi.org/10.1186/s12913-020-05821-2.

Pedersen, Morten Axel, Kristoffer Albris, and Nick Seaver. 2021. "The Political Economy of Attention." *Annual Review of Anthropology* 50 (1): 309–325. https://doi.org/10.1146/annurev-anthro-101819-110356.

Petrement, Simone. 1977. *Simone Weil: A Life*. Translated by Raymond Rosenthal. New York: Pantheon Books.

Petryna, Adriana. 2013. *Life Exposed: Biological Citizens after Chernobyl*. Reprint, Princeton, NJ: Princeton University Press.

Petryna, Adriana, and Karolina Follis. 2015. "Risks of Citizenship and Fault Lines of Survival." *Annual Review of Anthropology* 44 (1): 401–417. https://doi.org/10.1146/annurev-anthro-102313-030329.

Pines, Jesse M., Joshua A. Hilton, Ellen J. Weber, Annechien J. Alkemade, Hasan Al Shabanah, Philip D. Anderson, Michael Bernhard, et al. 2011. "International Perspectives on Emergency Department Crowding." *Academic Emergency Medicine: Official Journal of the Society for Academic Emergency Medicine* 18 (12): 1358–1370. https://doi.org/10.1111/j.1553-2712.2011.01235.x.

Pizza, Giovanni, and Andrea Ravenda. 2016. "Esperienza Dell'attesa e Retoriche Del Tempo." *Antropologia pubblica* 2 (1): 29–46. https://doi.org/10.1473/anpub.v2i1.17.

Pols, Jeannette. 2005. "Enacting Appreciations: Beyond the Patient Perspective." *Health Care Analysis* 13 (3): 203–221. https://doi.org/10.1007/s10728-005-6448

Porcellana, Valentina. 2022. *Antropologia del welfare: La cultura dei diritti sociali in Italia.* Ogliastro Cilento (Salerno): Licosia.

Portale Statistico AGENAS. (n.d.). Accessed 28 December 2024. https://stat.agenas.it/web/index.php?r=public%2Findex&report=23

Porter, Dorothy. 2011. "Health Citizenship: Essays in Social Medicine and Biomedical Politics." November. https://escholarship.org/uc/item/9ww2j8q1.

Raffaetà, Roberta. 2020. "Another Day in Dystopia: Italy in the Time of COVID-19." *Medical Anthropology* 39 (5): 371–373. https://doi.org/10.1080/01459740.2020.1746300.

Ramacciati, Nicola, Alessio Gili, Andrea Mezzetti, Andrea Ceccagnoli, Beniamino Addey, and Laura Rasero. 2019. "Violence towards Emergency Nurses: The 2016 Italian National Survey—a Cross-Sectional Study." *Journal of Nursing Management* 27 (4): 792–805. https://doi.org/10.1111/jonm.12733.

Redfield, Peter. 2013. *Life in Crisis: The Ethical Journey of Doctors without Borders.* Berkeley: University of California Press.

Rhodes, Lorna A. 1991. *Emptying Beds: The Work of an Emergency Psychiatric Unit.* 1st ed. Berkeley: University of California Press.

Riccio, Bruno. 2007. *"Toubab" e "Vu cumprà": Transnazionalità e rappresentazioni nelle migrazioni senegalesi in Italia.* Padua: Cooperativa Libraria Editrice Università di Padova.

———. 2019. *Mobilità: Incursioni etnografiche.* Milan: Mondadori Università.

Rowe, Rosemary, and Michael Calnan. 2006. "Trust Relations in Health Care: Developing a Theoretical Framework for the 'New' NHS." *Journal of Health Organization and Management* 20 (5): 376–396.

Saiani, Luisa. 2016. "La storia italiana della formazione infermieristica: La 'lunga marcia' dalle scuole regionali ai corsi di laurea magistrale." *TUTOR: An International, Peer Reviewed, Open Access Journal on Medical Education and Practice* 16 (1): 32–39. https://doi.org/10.14601/Tutor-18186.

Saines, J. C. 1999. "Violence and Aggression in A & E: Recommendations for Action." *Accident and Emergency Nursing* 7 (1): 8–12.

Schegloff, Emanuel A. 1997. "Whose Text? Whose Context?" *Discourse and Society* 8 (2): 165–187.

Scheper-Hughes, Nancy. 1993. *Death without Weeping: The Violence of Everyday Life in Brazil.* New ed. Berkeley: University of California Press.

———. 2003. "Rotten Trade: Millennial Capitalism, Human Values and Global Justice in Organs Trafficking." *Journal of Human Rights* 2 (2): 197–226. https://doi.org/10.1080/14754 83032000078189.

Scherer, Martin, Dagmar Lühmann, Agata Kazek, Heike Hansen, and Ingmar Schäfer. 2017. "Patients Attending Emergency Departments." *Deutsches Ärzteblatt International* 114 (39): 645–652. https://doi.org/10.3238/arztebl.2017.0645.

Schirripa, Pino. 2012. *Terapie religiose: Neoliberismo, cura, cittadinanza nel pentecostalismo contemporaneo.* Rome: CISU.

Schramm, Katharina, and Claire Beaudevin. 2019. "Sorting, Typing, Classifying." *Medicine Anthropology Theory* 6 (4). https://doi.org/10.17157/mat.6.4.767.

Schroer, Markus. 2019. "Sociology of Attention: Fundamental Reflections on a Theoretical Program." In *The Oxford Handbook of Cognitive Sociology*, edited by Wayne H. Brekhus and Gabe Ignatow, 425–447. Oxford: Oxford University Press.

Schweiger, Gottfried. 2020. "Absolute Poverty in European Welfare States." In *Dimensions of Poverty: Measurement, Epistemic Injustices, Activism*, edited by Valentin Beck, Henning Hahn, and Robert Lepenies, 163–176. Philosophy and Poverty. Cham, Switzerland: Springer. https://doi.org/10.1007/978-3-030-31711-9-10.

Seim, Josh. 2020. *Bandage, Sort, and Hustle: Ambulance Crews on the Front Lines of Urban Suffering*. 1st ed. Berkeley: University of California Press.

Seim, Josh, and Anthony DiMario. 2023. "City of Gauze: Medicine and the Governance of Urban Poverty." *Social Problems*, August 25, spad041. https://doi.org/10.1093/socpro/spad041.

Seligman, Adam B. 2000. *The Problem of Trust*. Princeton, NJ: Princeton University Press.

Sharp, Lesley A. 2013. *The Transplant Imaginary: Mechanical Hearts, Animal Parts, and Moral Thinking in Highly Experimental Science*. 1st ed. Berkeley: University of California Press.

Shore, David A. 2006. *The Trust Crisis in Healthcare: Causes, Consequences, and Cures*. Oxford: Oxford University Press.

Sidnell, Jack. 2010. *Conversation Analysis: An Introduction*. 1st ed. Chichester, UK: Wiley-Blackwell.

Sinclair, Douglas. 2007. "Emergency Department Overcrowding—Implications for Paediatric Emergency Medicine." *Paediatrics and Child Health* 12 (6): 491–494. https://doi.org/10.1093/pch/12.6.491.

Smith, Carole. 2005. "Understanding Trust and Confidence: Two Paradigms and Their Significance for Health and Social Care." *Journal of Applied Philosophy* 22 (3): 299–316. https://doi.org/10.1111/j.1468-5930.2005.00312.x.

Solomon, Harris. 2017. "Shifting Gears: Triage and Traffic in Urban India." *Medical Anthropology Quarterly* 31 (3): 349–364. https://doi.org/10.1111/maq.12367.

———. 2022. *Lifelines: The Traffic of Trauma*. Durham, NC: Duke University Press.

Sontag, Susan. 1988. *Illness as Metaphor*. Reprint, New York: Farrar, Straus and Giroux.

Star, Susan Leigh. 1999. "The Ethnography of Infrastructure." *American Behavioral Scientist* (Thousand Oaks) 43 (3): 377–391.

Star, Susan Leigh, and Karen Ruhleder. 1996. "Steps toward an Ecology of Infrastructure: Design and Access for Large Information Spaces." *Information Systems Research* 7 (1): 111–134.

Stevenson, Lisa. 2014. *Life Beside Itself: Imagining Care in the Canadian Arctic*. 1st ed. Oakland: University of California Press.

Stewart, Kathleen. 2007. *Ordinary Affects*. Durham, NC: Duke University Press.

Stonington, Scott. 2020. *The Spirit Ambulance: Choreographing the End of Life in Thailand*. 1st ed. Oakland: University of California Press.

Strathern, Marilyn. 2000. *Audit Cultures: Anthropological Studies in Accountability, Ethics and the Academy*. 1st ed. London: Routledge.

Strauss, Anselm L. 1978. *Negotiations: Varieties, Contexts, Processes and Social Order*. 1st ed. San Francisco: Jossey-Bass.

Street, Alice. 2011a. "Affective Infrastructure: Hospital Landscapes of Hope and Failure." *Space and Culture* 15 (1). https://doi.org/10.1177/1206331211426061.

———. 2011b. "Artefacts of Not-Knowing: The Medical Record, the Diagnosis and the Production of Uncertainty in Papua New Guinean Biomedicine." *Social Studies of Science* 41 (6): 815–834. https://doi.org/10.1177/0306312711419974.

————. 2012. "Seen by the State: Bureaucracy, Visibility and Governmentality in a Papua New Guinean Hospital." *Australian Journal of Anthropology* 23 (1): 1–21. https://doi.org/10.1111/j.1757-6547.2012.00164.x.

————. 2014. *Biomedicine in an Unstable Place: Infrastructure and Personhood in a Papua New Guinean Hospital.* Durham, NC: Duke University Press.

————. 2018. "Ghostly Ethics." *Medical Anthropology* 37 (8): 703–707. https://doi.org/10.1080/01459740.2018.1521400.

Street, Alice, and Simon Coleman. 2012. "Introduction: Real and Imagined Spaces." *Space and Culture* 15 (1): 4–17. https://doi.org/10.1177/1206331211421852.

Tarì, Marcello, and Ilaria Vanni. 2005. "On the Life and Deeds of San Precario, Patron Saint of Precarious Workers and Lives." *Fibreculture Journal*, no. 5 (January). https://five.fibreculturejournal.org/fcj-023-on-the-life-and-deeds-of-san-precario-patron-saint-of-precarious-workers-and-lives/.

Throop, C. Jason, and Alessandro Duranti. 2015. "Attention, Ritual Glitches, and Attentional Pull: The President and the Queen." *Phenomenology and the Cognitive Sciences* 14 (4): 1055–1082. https://doi.org/10.1007/s11097-014-9397-4.

Throop, C. Jason, and Keith M. Murphy. 2002. "Bourdieu and Phenomenology: A Critical Assessment." *Anthropological Theory* 2 (2): 185–207. https://doi.org/10.1177/1469962002002002630.

Ticktin, Miriam I. 2011. *Casualties of Care: Immigration and the Politics of Humanitarianism in France.* 1st ed. Berkeley: University of California Press.

Tronto, Joan. 1987. "Beyond Gender Difference to a Theory of Care." *Signs* 12 (4): 644–663.

————. 1994. *Moral Boundaries.* 1st ed. New York: Routledge.

Trundle, Catherine. 2020. "Tinkering Care, State Responsibility, and Abandonment: Nuclear Test Veterans and the Mismatched Temporalities of Justice in Claims for Health Care." *Anthropology and Humanism* 45 (2): 202–211.

Tsing, Anna Lowenhaupt. 2015. *The Mushroom at the End of the World: On the Possibility of Life in Capitalist Ruins.* Princeton, NJ: Princeton University Press.

Varley, Emma, and Saiba Varma. 2018. "Spectral Ties: Hospital Hauntings across the Line of Control." *Medical Anthropology* 37 (8): 630–644.

Varma, Saiba. 2020. *The Occupied Clinic: Militarism and Care in Kashmir.* Durham, NC: Duke University Press.

Vassy, Carine. 2001. "Categorisation and Micro-Rationing: Access to Care in a French Emergency Department." *Sociology of Health and Illness* 23 (5): 615–632. https://doi.org/10.1111/1467-9566.00268.

Wahlberg, Ayo. 2009. "Serious Disease as Kinds of Living." In *Contested Categories: Life Sciences in Society,* edited by Susanne Bauer and Ayo Wahlberg, 89–112. London: Routledge. https://doi.org/10.4324/9781315573977-6.

Wahlberg, Ayo, and Nikolas Rose. 2015. "The Governmentalization of Living: Calculating Global Health." *Economy and Society* 44 (1): 60–90. https://doi.org/10.1080/03085147.2014.983830.

Wamsiedel, Marius. 2018. "Reasonableness: Legitimate Reasons for Illegitimate Presentations at the ED." *Sociology of Health and Illness* 40 (8): 1347–1360. https://doi.org/10.1111/1467-9566.12776.

Wendland, Claire L. 2010. *A Heart for the Work: Journeys through an African Medical School.* 1st ed. Chicago: University of Chicago Press.

WHO (World Health Organization). n.d. "Innovative Care for Chronic Conditions: Building Blocks for Action." Accessed 30 September 2019. https://www.who.int/publications/i/item/innovative-care-for-chronic-conditions-building-blocks-for-actions

Whyte, Susan Reynolds, Sjaak van der Geest, and Anita Hardon. 2003. *Social Lives of Medi-cines*. 1st ed. Cambridge: Cambridge University Press.

Williamson, Amelia, and Barbara Hoggart. 2005. "Pain: A Review of Three Commonly Used Pain Rating Scales." *Journal of Clinical Nursing* 14 (7): 798–804. https://doi.org/10.1111/j .1365-2702.2005.01121.x.

Wind, Gitte. 2008. "Negotiated Interactive Observation: Doing Fieldwork in Hospital Set-tings." *Anthropology and Medicine* 15 (2): 79–89.

Yanagisako, Sylvia Junko. 2002. *Producing Culture and Capital: Family Firms in Italy*. Prince-ton, NJ: Princeton University Press.

Zink, Brian J. 2005. *Anyone, Anything, Anytime: A History of Emergency Medicine*. Philadelphia: Elsevier Health Sciences.

INDEX

ABOUT THE AUTHOR

MIRKO PASQUINI is an assistant professor in medical anthropology at the School of Global Studies at the University of Gothenburg and an affiliated researcher at the Centre for Medical Humanities at Uppsala University in Sweden. His research interests combine hospital ethnography and primary care in Italy and Sweden, with a focus on health inequalities, health care governance, the social dynamics of attention, violence, and trust and mistrust in care interactions. His work has appeared in the *Lancet*, in *Medical Anthropology*, and in *Global Public Health and Human Organization*, among other international journals. Mirko Pasquini is also part of the editorial board of *Lancet* Cases in Global Social Medicine. Since 2018, he has been engaged in health workers' training in structural competency, an innovative curriculum in social medicine in Sweden, Denmark, and Italy.

Available titles in the Medical Anthropology: Health, Inequality, and Social Justice series: